£6.95
P

DEATH, BRAIN DEATH AND ETHICS

DAVID LAMB

CROOM HELM
London & Sydney

Croom Helm Ltd, Provident House, Burrell Row,
Beckenham, Kent, BR3 1AT
Croom Helm Australia, 44-50 Waterloo Road,
North Ryde, 2113, New South Wales
New in paperback 1988

British Library Cataloguing in Publication Data
Lamb, David
    Death, brain death and ethics.
    1. Death — Moral and ethical aspects
    I. Title
    174'.24   R725.5
    ISBN 0-7099-4184-6

Printed and bound in Great Britain
by Billing & Sons Limited, Worcester.

CONTENTS

ACKNOWLEDGEMENTS

This book has grown out of a series of lectures and seminars in Ethics and Advanced Philosophy of Science at the University of Manchester, England, and out of papers read at philosophy meetings at the universities of Southampton, Sussex and Manchester. I am grateful to participants at these meetings for their helpful comments and suggestions. I would also like to thank Hilary Walford, who on behalf of Croom Helm gave valuable assistance in the preparation of this book for publication. A special note of gratitude is owed to Dr Christopher Pallis of the Royal Postgraduate Medical School, University of London. I have benefited considerably from conversation with him over many years and from his constructive advice and criticism. The usual disclaimers apply.

PREFACE

This book examines the concept of death against the background of dramatic changes in medical technology. Developments in resuscitation techniques and the ability of machines to take over such vital functions as spontaneous breathing challenge traditional ways of diagnosing death. As a result physicians have employed brain-related criteria in certain cases where vital processes are being maintained by artificial means. While tests for the death of the brain are continually improving very little work has been done to explain why the death of the brain is a necessary and sufficient condition for the death of a human being. In fact, the very concept of 'brain death' has remained unclear in most of the medical literature related to this subject. Is brain death a new concept of death? Is it a new set of criteria for diagnosing death? Does it imply an alternative definition of death? It is clear that the term has arisen in the context of modern medical science but how does it stand in relation to older accounts of death? Can brain death be defined? Some philosophers have argued that it should not be defined, but left undetermined.

These questions are examined in a survey of recent literature on the definition and diagnosis of death. It will be argued that brain death can be precisely defined and determined and that a biological concept of death, such as brain death, can be given a philosophical foundation. The book examines traditional criteria for death and various new formulations of the concept of death in both medical and philosophical texts. Definitions of brain death — some of which have become statute law — are critically examined. In addition to the conceptual and philosophical issues related to such definitions the book also examines ethical and social-policy questions which arise out of attempts to redefine the boundaries of life.

This book has been written for lay-readers, ethicists, philosophers and even physicians who may be stimulated by a discussion of some of the philosophical beliefs which underlie their clinical practice. The objective is primarily philosophical, that is to say, arguments are not introduced to corroborate or refute current practice but to clarify its underlying concepts, and thus emphasise how philosophical and practical matters interrelate.

David Lamb
Manchester

1 INTRODUCTION

There is no such thing as a natural death: nothing that happens to a man is ever natural, since his presence calls the world into question. All men must die: but for every man his death is an accident and, even if he knows it, and consents to it, an unjustified violation.

Simone de Beauvoir, *A Very Easy Death*.

Is death an illness to be conquered, like polio, or cancer or syphilis? Or is its meaning quite different? Wittgenstein says that death is not an event in life. Among other things this means that death is unknowable, beyond the scope of scientific evidence. The concept of death, unlike that of disease, has a significance that extends beyond scientific knowledge and clinical practice. It is central to most of the great religions and is given a special role in ethical discourse. In many cultures death is seen as a natural and inevitable end to life. When the time of death approaches, the traditional task of the physician is to render comfort and assistance to the patient in his or her remaining hours. But in the West death is increasingly seen as an enemy to be combated. This is a consequence of the influence of scientific medicine and is a relatively recent phenomenon. Whereas physicians formerly accepted death as natural but strove to eliminate disease, in recent years the very idea of death has come to resemble a disease to be eliminated. This change of attitudes has led to a shift of emphasis in theoretical and practical questions associated with death. For the Greeks and early Chinese the acceptance of death as a natural event meant that questions could be posed regarding the possibility of some kind of life after death. In a more secular age we are more concerned with the mechanics of death, its postponement and possible reversal.

This book is primarily concerned with philosophical and ethical problems arising out of attempts to define the end points of human life. For this reason it will be necessary to examine a wide range of questions which invariably transcend the traditional boundaries between philosophy and medicine.

Philosophical questions concerning the meaning of life and death will be examined in Chapter 2. Closely related to this topic is the question 'What is considered so essential to human life such that when it is

1

lost we consider the individual dead?' This question underlies the inquiry in Chapters 3, 4, 5 and 8. Clinical questions – such as 'What are the best technical methods for diagnosing the death of a human being?' – will be dealt with in Chapter 6. The question of whether a clear-cut moment of death can be determined will be considered in Chapter 7. The ethical implications of the acceptance of brain-related criteria for death will be considered in Chapters 9 and 10.

Legal-policy questions – which take the form of asking 'When should the law and the courts regard a person as dead?' and 'When should the medical profession be authorised to pronounce a person dead?' – are outside the scope of this text. It will be maintained, however, that the courts should accept that a person can be pronounced dead when clinical criteria, based on a clearly defined concept of brain death, have been met. It might be noted in this context that the medical profession has no inherent authority to define or determine death. This authority is granted by law. Occasionally the law does not rely on medical expertise when determining death, as in cases where the courts decide that someone is 'missing presumed dead'.

Although the definition of death is not an exclusively medical matter, and may be influenced by religious, legal or political criteria, the concepts and criteria examined here will be those familiar to physicians. Inherent in any medically grounded definition is the assumption that death is an irreversible state, which can be diagnosed in terms of the cessation of crucial cardio-respiratory and neural functions. Normally it is assumed that death takes place at a specific moment, although from a biological standpoint death can be considered as a more gradual process.

If an irreversible loss is central to the concept of death it follows that if a patient recovers after being pronounced dead it should not be said that 'he was dead and is now alive again', but that, contrary to all appearances, he was alive all the time. It may be objected that this claim rests on a rather limited resort to the linguistic practices of contemporary medicine. In many other spheres of discourse, notably religion, there are accounts of the reversibility of death. There are frequent accounts in the media of patients being 'brought back to life'. Such reports, however, must be discounted, since they amount to little more than dramatic cures or resuscitation in cases where the indices of persistent life were not always very obvious. Such cases usually involve cardiac arrest followed by temporary suspension of respiration. Experienced physicians would not accept them as examples of the reversibility of death. Graphic accounts of experiences in the 'next world' are merely highly dramatised ways of saying that consciousness was temporarily lost during an episode of cardiac arrest. Nevertheless these accounts have been given a religious significance encouraged by dramatic reporting in the media of experiences 'beyond the veil'. All of this might suggest that, for many people, death is not perceived as inevitably irreversible but is relative to the exponents of scientific medicine. In this respect the analytic relationship between 'knowing that P is dead' and 'P being dead' might be said to hold only for the specialist in medicine. But if this were the case, the conceptual foundations of contemporary medicine would seem to be in conflict with the fundamental claims of most of the major religions. For in both primitive cultures and classical antiquity, as well as in contemporary religious movements, there exist deeply held beliefs that death does not mean total extinction. In many cultures death is seen in terms of a journey. Food is often provided to assist the traveller on his or her way 'beyond death'.

Yet none of this actually contradicts the medical assertion of the irreversibility of death. Although religious practices may refer to the conquest and reversibility of death, many elaborate funeral rites indicate a recognition of the grandeur of death and stress the significance and worth of the life that has passed away, rather than the superstitious prediction of unlimited life extension. For ceremonial purposes a corpse may be spoken of as a being with mortal attributes, but is nevertheless recognised as a corpse. Food may be left for the use of the departed on his journey to the next world, but no one has ever expected the corpse to consume it. And if the food were actually eaten it would indicate, to religious believer and to physician alike, that the 'deceased' was still alive. Moreover, the practice of leaving food for the dead has never been abandoned despite massive evidence that corpses have never availed themselves of it. All of this suggests that religious accounts of survival after death do not contradict clinical evidence for the cessation of integrated life. That death is an irreversible interruption of physical continuity is not disputed by either medicine or religion.

Although several religious theories assert that life continues after the separation of the soul from the body, it is extremely difficult to conceptualise this continued existence. Fortunately, it is not necessary to do so. Religious concepts of the transcendence of death only appear to contradict known medical concepts of death. Whilst theologians may hold that the soul survives bodily dissolution, there is no disagreement over the ordinary use of the term 'dead'. A person pronounced dead by a competent physician, according to clearly defined criteria, is no more expected to 'recover' for the theist than for the secularist.

In order systematically to analyse the concept of death being dis-cussed by modern medicine it is necessary to distinguish between *syste-mic death* (or death as traditionally understood) and *brain death*. Systemic death is death defined by conventional means, i.e., in terms of irreversible cessation of cardio-respiratory function. Brain death has been defined as the 'total and irreversible dysfunction . . . of all neuronal components of the intracranial cavity, that is, both cerebral hemispheres, brainstem and cerebellum.' (Korein, 1978, p.21) Through-out the following chapters the concept of brain death will be outlined in greater detail and defended against criticism. It will also be argued that cardio-respiratory arrest is only a mechanism for causing brain death and that it is only lethal if it lasts long enough for certain critical areas of the brain to die.

The concept of brain death emerged in France in 1959. Since then hundreds, perhaps thousands, of patients throughout the world have been diagnosed as brain dead, maintained on ventilators and observed until their hearts stopped. The term *'coma dépassé'* (literally a state beyond coma) was coined by French neurologists to describe a condi-tion of irreversible coma associated with irreversible loss of the capacity to breathe. The patients had all sustained massive, irreversibly, struc-tural brain damage. They were totally unresponsive, apnoeic (unable to breathe spontaneously) and had no detectable electrophysiological activity in either the superficial or deeper parts of their brain. Provided their breathing was immediately taken over by a machine, their hearts could be kept going for a short while.

Patients in *coma dépassé* had not only lost all capacity to respond to external stimuli, they could not even cope with their internal milieu; they were poikilothermic, had diabetes insipidus and could not sustain their own blood pressure. The cardiac prognosis of this condition was at most a few days, but sometimes as little as a few hours. (Pallis, 1983, b, p.34) Outside France the term *'coma dépassé'* never really caught on. The condition was of course encountered wherever resuscitation was sufficiently well organised, and intensive care units were sufficiently well equipped, to prevent irreversible apnoea immediately resulting in cessation of cardiac action. Following the publication in 1968 of a re-port of the 'Ad Hoc Committee of the Harvard Medical School to Examine the Definition of Brain Death', the condition of *brain death* (which was exactly what the French had described as *'coma dépassé'*) achieved world-wide recognition. In the years following the publication of the Harvard Report it gradually became realised that the essential components or 'physiological kernel' of brain death was death of the brainstem (*brainstem death*). The brainstem contains (in its upper part) crucial centres responsible for generating the capacity for consciousness. In its lower part it contains the respiratory centre. It is death of the brainstem (nearly always the result of increased intracranial pressure) which produces the crucial signs (apnoeic coma) which doctors detect at the bedside, when they diagnose brain death.

The last twenty years have seen the gradual acceptance of the proposition that the death of the brain is a necessary and sufficient condition for the death of the individual. The last ten years have seen a parallel development: the gradual realisation that death of the brainstem is the necessary and sufficient condition for death of the brain as a whole – and that brainstem death is therefore itself synonymous with the death of the individual. This latter realisation first received implicit recognition in statements issued by the Conference of Medical Royal Colleges and Their Faculties in 1976 and 1979. Proponents of brainstem criteria for death argue that death of the brainstem is itself death (a philosophical position that will be developed further in this book). They also point out that a diagnosis of brainstem death has in every observed case been followed by eventual circulatory arrest (an empirical observation). Brainstem death, it is argued, is the 'point of no return' in the process of dying, the stage at which 'loss of integration' becomes irreversible.

The clearly interrelated conditions of whole brain death and brainstem death should not be confused with another, very different, condition in which massive brain damage is largely confined to the cerebral hemispheres, sparing much of the brainstem and in particular the capacity to breathe spontaneously. Such patients have usually been the victims of severe head injury or of massive anoxic insults to the brain (lack of oxygen wrecks the cerebral hemispheres before it damages the brainstem). These individuals are said to be in a *persistent vegetative state* (Jennett and Plum, 1972) or to suffer from neocortical death. Institutions for the chronic sick all over the world are full of such patients. It is important, both scientifically and ethically, to avoid confusing brain death with such non-cognitive states. Patients in persistent vegetative states display no evidence of self-awareness and exhibit no purposeful responses to external stimuli. Their eyes are periodically open, and they show sleep-wake sequences. They may exhibit yawning or chewing movements and may swallow spontaneously. A variety of simple or complex reflex responses may be elicited from them. Unlike whole brain death or brainstem death (which signify death of the organism as a whole and have a cardiac prognosis numbered in hours or days), the persistent vegetative state has a potential cardiac prognosis of months or years. The longest recorded survivor in this state was Elaine Eposito, who lapsed into such a condition following surgery on August 6, 1941 and died 37 years later on November 25, 1978. (McWhirter, 1981) Closely related to the vegetative state are patients with various severe congenital malformations of the brain. These patients are not dead either. They too may live for years.

The terms 'cerebral death' and 'irreversible coma' are best avoided altogether, as they have been loosely used, in the past, to refer to both whole brain death and the persistent vegetative state.

When terms like 'brain death' and 'vegetative state' are used as if they were synonymous (in proposals for euthanasia or termination of treatment) there is not only factual error but serious risk of ethical abuse. Patients in a vegetative state are not dead. No culture in the world would consider them as fit for burial, organ removal, experimentation, etc. The arguments in Chapters 5 and 10 which seek to exclude these states from the definition of death will only be directed at philosophers, and their non-philosophical imitators in the media, who still seem prone to such confusion.

Before developments and refinements in brain-related criteria, death was usually determined in terms of the irreversible loss of cardiovascular and respiratory activity. However, developments in resuscitation technology and transplantation techniques have revealed inadequacies in traditional concepts of death. When a dead person's heart can beat in the chest of a living person whose own heart has been removed from his or her body and discarded then the significance of one's heartbeat as a determinant of life is lost. It is clear that the concept of brain death reflects a shift of opinion in response to technological intervention. Consequently, it has been asked whether brain death is really equivalent to the death of the person. Now the concept of personal identity is very vague, and criteria for its loss is a subject of philosophical controversy and prone to constant redefinition. The relationship between brain death and personal identity will be examined in Chapter 8, where it is argued that, if the definition of death were based on concepts of the non-survival of the person, it would be subject to constant redefinition and uncertainty. Against this it is necessary to point out that the death of a human being is too serious a matter for scepticism to obtain a foothold. A clearly defined concept of death is therefore necessitated on both scientific and ethical grounds. For this reason a biological concept of death will be proposed and defended which will not be exclusively dependent upon consciousness and personhood, but on criteria which indicate an irreversible loss of essential integrative functions. (These include generating the capacity for consciousness; alerting; varying the blood pressure in response to changes in cardiac rate; varying the cardiac rate in response to changes in blood pressure, and varying the respiratory rate in response to changing concentrations of CO_2 etc.) The loss of these central functions it will be argued, is a point in the process of dying beyond classical philosophical criteria for loss of personhood. A person may be said to have died on a number of levels; physically, psychologically, morally or spiritually. On the other hand the death of a human being is definite; a matter of scientific fact.

In Chapters 2, 3, 4 and 5 it will be argued that death of the brainstem provides both a necessary and a sufficient definition of the death of a human being, in that it provides a physiological substratum for the 'irreversible loss of function of the organism as a whole'. Other concepts of death, including those based on death of the cerebral hemispheres or on social or moral criteria, are, it will be argued, both scientifically and ethically unwarranted. Death is primarily a biological phenomenon. The death of a man is no different from the death of a dog or cat. In all cases the brain is the critical system, and brainstem function its vital ingredient. Essential to the concept of brain death is the belief in the existence of a single vital system whose irreversible loss is synonymous with the death of the organism as a whole. As Korein (1978, p. 20) points out, 'the premise underlying the concept of brain death is that there is a single critical vital system, the brain, whose irreversible destruction is both a necessary and sufficient condition in considering an individual as dead.' This statement rests on a large mass of clinical and experimental observations indicating that the essence of the human organism, including both internal and external behaviour, is subserved by the brain, which is irreplaceable. (ibid., p. 20)

At what stage is the brain dead? When every neuron has been destroyed? Or when a critical mass of neurons at a critical site have been destroyed, thus rendering the remainder dysfunctional? It will be argued in Chapter 4 that the brain as a whole is dead when a critical mass of neurons is destroyed. This critical mass is the brainstem. The minimum requirements for human life are the *capacity* for consciousness and the *capacity* for respiration and heartbeat. These are, respectively, upper and lower brainstem functions.

Criteria for the diagnosis of brain death are being continually refined by clinical and experimental research. Yet confusion persists partly because of the use of ambiguous terms like 'irreversible coma' and 'cerebral death', and partly because people confuse questions related to the determination of death with other tangentially related problems. It is most important to avoid confusing the identification of brain death with (1) criteria for diagnosing the vegetative state; (2) questions concerning then need for cadaver transplants; (3) cost-benefit arguments related to the employment of artificial life-support systems; (4) decisions to terminate artificial life support, with a view to facilitating various forms of 'allowing to die'.

A diagnosis of brain death must never be confused with concerns about the quality of residual life in vegetative states. Moreover a shortage of transplant organs should not be met by changing criteria for diagnosing death, or by the adoption of more lenient or flexible standards. Only when a human being is dead, according to criteria derived from a well-grounded concept of death, should consideration be given to the removal of usable organs. Similarly, questions concerning a patient's right to terminate treatment and requests for accelerated death have nothing to do with a clinical diagnosis of death. Neither moral, religious nor cost-benefit considerations should be allowed to blur the crucial distinction between a decision as to when death has occurred and a decision as to whether a death is to be allowed to occur.

2   DEATH: CONCEPT AND CRITERIA

'To give a new concept' can only mean to introduce a new employment of a concept, a new practice.

'Concept' is a vague concept.
                L. Wittgenstein, *Remarks on the Foundations of Mathematics*

Introduction

In this chapter the relationship between the philosophical aspects of
death and the clinical requirements for a diagnosis of death will be
examined. In the first section, 'Understanding Death', these conceptual
and practical aspects will be addressed in the context of a proposed
definition of death as 'the irreversible loss of function of the organism
as a whole'. It will be maintained that this definition is only applicable
in the context of brain-related criteria for death. The second section of
this chapter, 'Understanding Brain Death', will examine the philosophical status of brain death.

Understanding Death

Unlike the concept of disease, the concept of death cannot be exclusively determined by medical criteria. This is because it is related to
more general philosophical beliefs concerning the *meaning* of life and
death. Yet the fact that clinical considerations regarding the concept
and criteria of death, and related tests, should be and are primarily
influenced by philosophical considerations is scarcely recognised in
medical literature. It is true that some philosophers and physicians
believe that the determination of death is primarily a task for the
medical community, but, as High (1972, p. 456) has pointed out, this is
to ignore the fact that essential philosophical questions cannot be
reduced to the sciences of biology and medicine:

If a philosopher or lawyer or theologian wants to claim that he has
no professional business with the issue and that it is a purely medical

9

or biological one, that too, I suggest, is to opt for a philosophical position concerning the concept of death, namely, that it is empirically decidable.

It may be wise to decide that the medical profession is best equipped to determine whether or not death has occurred, but such a preference is primarily philosophical. As a rule, the more one believes that philosophical presuppositions have been avoided, the less rigorous will be those presuppositions.

Death has been legally defined as the absence of life, but the concept of life is rarely, if ever, defined. The *Shorter Oxford English Dictionary* is unhelpful; it defines death as 'the final cessation of the vital function of an animal or plant', 'the loss or cessation of life in a part'. At this level of generality it is not immediately clear where the concept of death stands. Not only is the definition of death rather elusive, but the very meaning of definition in this context is highly ambiguous. Many neurological definitions of death are purely operational, based on matters of medical fact and clinical diagnosis, and might involve arguments about whether or not the electroencelphalogram (EEG) is relevant. This may be distinguished from discussions over the definition of death in a religious and philosophical setting, where questions concerning the meaning and significance of life are examined. Whilst the technical expertise of physicians may be employed in a diagnosis of death, the definition of death embraces broader philosophical considerations such as the meaning and value of life and the point of existence.

It has been argued that physicians *qua* physicians have no special expertise in these philosophical problems and can deal only with technical questions relating to the conditions in which human beings display vital signs. Capron and Kass (1980, p. 47) distinguish sharply between medical and extra-medical judgements when they argue, for example, that physicians can show that a person may exhibit

'total unawareness to externally applied stimuli and inner need and complete unresponsiveness', and they may predict that when tests for this condition yield the same results over a twenty-four hour period there is only a very minute chance that the coma will ever be 'reversed'. Yet the judgement that 'total unawareness . . . and complete unresponsiveness' are salient characteristics of death, or that a certain level of risk of error is acceptable, requires more than technical expertise and goes beyond medical authority, properly understood.

But whilst it is important to separate the sphere of the philosophical from the medical, it is equally important to stress that in any discussion of death neither party can afford to ignore the contributions of the other. Medical judgements are informed by philosophical presuppositions, whether or not the latter are explicitly formulated. The diagnosis of any illness may be clinical and empirical, but it would be lacking in significance if there were no underlying concepts of health and disease. Whether a patient is classified as dead or alive depends on our understanding of the relevant concept of death. According to Capron and Kass (1980) the departure from the traditional concept of death manifest in the employment of brain-related criteria has brought these extra-medical concepts to the forefront of concern. Whilst traditional criteria, based on the cessation of cardio-respiratory functions, remained congruent with public conceptions of death, the phenomenon of death remained exclusively a matter of medical concern. But once medicine appeared to depart from traditional criteria for determining death, clarification of these extra-medical concepts of death became a matter of urgent concern for those responsible for the management of death. In view of the importance attached to a diagnosis of death in terms of the social, religious, political and ethical consequences, it is essential that this challenge be met and that the concept of death be made explicit. Furthermore, it is essential that criteria and tests for death should be logically derived from the appropriate concept of death.

The concept of death involves a philosophical judgement that a significant change has taken place, which presupposes an idea of the necessary conditions of life. These may range from the faculties involved in social interaction to the capacity to maintain bodily integration. Concepts of death may vary according to cultural patterns, religious traditions and scientific practice. (Pallis, 1983a) They may include such distinct formulations as 'the separation of soul and body', 'destruction of all physical structures', 'loss of the capacity for social interaction', 'irreversible loss of consciousness', 'loss of bodily integration', and many others. Related to these concepts are appropriate criteria, and tests to ascertain that the criteria have been met. It follows that any shift in the concept of death will necessitate corresponding changes in the criteria and tests for death. However, it does not follow that new criteria and tests mean that a change of concept has taken place. They may indicate nothing more than refinements of previous criteria and tests. For example, the employment of stethoscopes and cardiograms constituted technically better tests for death which did not entail any departure from the traditional cardio-respiratory-based concept of death.

Criteria for death only have meaning if they can be shown to be logically derived from the appropriate concept of death. It is therefore meaningless to use 'free-floating criteria' which are not derived from a clearly-determined concept of death. (Browne, 1983, and Pallis's critique, 1983b) Clarity concerning the concept of death provides a point of reference when deciding upon criteria, but some definitions of death are philosophically inadequate despite the fact that criteria can be logically derived from them. Consequently an investigation of the philosophical basis of any concept of death is important, as we can see from the following example:

> In the Middle Ages, if one entered certain monasteries one ceased to enjoy the limited rights and heavy duties of the outside world. One would be considered 'dead' by civil society. The appropriate criteria for such a concept of death would presumably be a certificate from the Father Superior of the monastery confirming that one had entered it. Esoteric concepts may be met by esoteric criteria. (Pallis, 1983a, p. 2)

In so far as these criteria fulfilled this admittedly esoteric concept of death, there are no problems. But as a definition of death 'entering certain monastic orders in the Middle Ages' is wholly inadequate. Presuming that this definition is not held *within* the monastery, a person could be simultaneously dead and not dead, according to which concept of death was being applied. On leaving the monastery and returning to the outside world, he would be in an anomalous situation of experiencing a resurrection, and moreover one not preceded by death in any physical sense. If anomalies such as this are to be avoided, then a minimum requirement for an adequate concept of death must be that it entails physical destruction. Concepts of death, such as 'entering a monastery' or exclusion from the family, tribe or clan, are widely used and yield appropriate criteria. But they can refer to death only in a metaphorical sense.

The essential point here is that some concepts are more relevant than others. The requirement for a definition of death is a demand for the selection of a concept that is superior to others. For this reason vaguely formulated and indeterminate concepts should be eschewed. Thus a concept of death as 'the loss of that which is essentially significant to the nature of man' is unsatisfactory, since we can say that a patient has lost what is essentially significant but is still alive. This is because concepts like 'essentially significant' are by their very nature undetermined. For if by 'the loss of what is essentially significant' is meant 'the loss of the capacity for social interaction' then various interpretations are possible, from loss of libido to blindness, from senility to dementia, which will provide appropriate criteria. But the question of which, if any, of these states might best fulfil the requirements of the definition cannot be answered without further conceptual guidelines. On what grounds can it be inferred that 'massive brain damage', or 'loss of reproductive function' and so on amount to the 'loss of what is essentially significant'? Furthermore, all of the fore-mentioned criteria may be fulfilled when it is patently obvious that the patient is alive and, in some cases, that his situation is even reversible. If the 'loss of that which is essentially significant' is to have any meaning as a concept of death, then it must be framed so that it involves an irreversible state where the organism as a whole cannot function. Only a concept which specifies the irreversible loss of specified functions (due to the destruction of their anatomical substratum) can avoid the anomalous situation where a patient is said to be alive according to one concept but dead according to another. The only wholly satisfactory concept of death is that which trumps other concepts of death in so far as it yields a diagnosis of death which is beyond dispute. It follows that any criterion which, when fulfilled, leaves it possible for someone to say that the patient is still alive, is unsatisfactory. For this reason concepts relating specifically to psychological functions or moral qualities are wholly inadequate. In fact any criterion which, when fulfilled, leaves it possible for the organism as a whole to continue to function is inadequate. It should not be possible to say that the person is still alive although the criterion has been met, nor to say that the person is dead although the criterion has not been met.

Essential to any valid concept of death is the prediction of irreversibility. Criteria and tests must be so devised that, once the requirements of the definition have been satisfied, there can be no return, with or without mechanical assistance, to the organism's previous state. This position is entirely compatible with religious theories regarding existence after death, none of which would conflict with established physiological criteria and tests for death. One might adhere to a religious concept of death according to which death is characterised in terms of the separation of the soul from the body, but this does not entail any dispute with acceptable medical criteria for diagnosing the death of the organism as a whole. Although most religions reject the idea of the finality of death and interpret death as a transitional stage, it is nevertheless held to be an irreversible change (excepting miracles involving divine intervention), the onset of which is diagnosed by biologically based criteria.

The concept of death that will be proposed and defended in this chapter is the *'irreversible loss of function of the organism as a whole'*. There is confusion between this and 'death of the whole organism'. This is often present — although unformulated — in arguments which maintain that the concept of death should be left undetermined, or that death is a process with no special point at which a non-arbitrary diagnosis can be factually ascertained. (Browne, 1983) Criteria for the 'death of the whole organism' could only be met by tests for putrefaction, since cellular life in certain tissues can continue long after it has ceased in others, and long past the point where the organism as a whole has ceased to function. However, putrefaction has never been seriously advanced as a definition of death by either physicians or philosophers. Consequently, the argument that the concept of death should remain undetermined has no place in a world where practical decisions regarding the criteria of death necessitate an acceptable concept. In contrast criteria for 'irreversible loss of function of the organism as a whole' can be determined with precision, and appropriate diagnostic tests are constantly being developed. (see Pallis, 1983a) The 'irreversible loss of function of the organism as a whole' is a biological concept which yields clinical criteria and tests. It presupposes the irreversible loss of the capacity for consciousness and the irreversible loss of the capacity to breathe, and hence sustain a spontaneous heartbeat. It supersedes ethical and religious-based concepts and its appropriate criterion is the death of the critical system as measured by tests for the irreversible cessation of brainstem function.

Failure to understand the relationship between the concept and criteria for death may lead to serious errors of judgement in practical matters. A patient in a vegetative state, it is argued, may meet a concept of death as 'a worthless existence' but, unless the individual's critical system is dead, it will not satisfy the concept of death formulated above as the 'irreversible loss of function of the organism as a whole'. The latter concept is currently employed in medical practice, if not explicitly formulated. It explains why an anencephalic infant would not be regarded as dead as long as its brainstem remained intact. (Normally anencephalics only survive for a few hours, but a case has been reported of such a child, with no evidence of cognitive function, surviving under the total care of its mother for 17 years.) (Korein, 1978, p. 366) Confusion between the concept and criteria of death has been atrributed to the Harvard Committee's Report of 1968 (see Veatch, 1978a) which regarded 'irreversible coma' as equivalent to 'brain death' and then conflated irreversible coma with death. Nowhere did the Committee indicate how it had moved from a discussion of clinical criteria for a diagnosis of irreversible coma to the philosophical judgement that irreversible coma was death. It is one thing, argues Veatch, to diagnose irreversible coma, but another thing entirely to conclude that a patient in such a state is dead, or that the criteria for this state meet the concept of death. The very first sentence of the Harvard Report (Harvard Medical School, 1968) revealed this confusion. 'Our primary purpose', it stated, 'is to define irreversible coma as a new criterion of death,' which according to Veatch, (1978b, p. 307) the Report failed to offer any arguments or evidence to show that irreversible coma was synonymous with the death of the person as a whole. Whilst the Committee offered what it considered as 'empirically accurate predictors of irreversible coma', it did not as Veatch points out, 'deal at all with the more difficult question: "If a person is in irreversible coma, should he be treated as if he were dead?" '

For the above reasons it has become commonplace in the literature on brain death to describe the concept of death as a philosophical matter and the development of diagnostic criteria as a task for medical expertise and to warn against conflating definitions of what death is with the problem of when death occurs. The philosophical analysis of death is held to identify what it is that the diagnostic criteria are supposed to determine. (see Korein, 1978, Veatch, 1978a, 1978b)

Whilst this distinction is important, it is nevertheless equally important that it should not be drawn too rigidly. Philosophical issues do not exist in complete isolation from technical and scientific issues; they interact and interpenetrate. For this reason a more flexible distinction has been formulated by Bernat, Culver and Gert (1981, p. 389)

> Providing a definition is primarily a philosophical task: the choice of the criteria is primarily medical: and the selection of tests to prove that the criterion is satisfied is solely a medical matter.

This formulation can be illustrated as follows: suppose the concept of death were 'absence of fluid flow', then the criteria would be based on cessation of pulse, heartbeat and respiration, and could be determined by relatively straightforward empirical tests. If, however, the concept were the 'integrated functioning of the organism as a whole', one would have to decide which organ has decisive responsibility for this. If it is a matter of general agreement that the brain has this responsibility, then tests for measuring brain functions will be important. The formulation proposed by Bernat *et al.* has the merit of maintaining the distinction between philosophical discourse regarding the concept of death and medical discourse. Yet it recognises that, whilst philosophical and practical issues can be distinguished at one level, they mutually interact at another level. It is therefore important to be wary of attempts to settle — at the outset of any discussion — which kinds of problems belong exclusively to philosophy and which belong exclusively to medicine. Whilst Veatch's and Korein's formulations correctly identify the concept of death as a philosophical issue and the criteria for death as a practical matter, the three-level distinction between concept, criteria and practical tests, which is proposed by Bernat *et al.*, is preferable because it acknowledges the interaction between conceptual issues and the application of criteria in a practical context.

Understanding Brain Death

How can the concept of death be understood in terms of an interaction between conceptual issues and practical criteria? What is brain death? Is it a concept of death for philosophers to investigate or a name for a set of criteria employed by physicians? Is it a technical concept used by medical scientists in contrast to the loosely formulated concepts of death employed by laypersons? Moreover, is it a new concept of death, or a refinement of the traditional concept? And if it is a new concept, can it coexist with the traditional concept?

Is Brain Death a Concept of a Set of Criteria?

Korein (1978, p. 20) defines brain death as a concept of death according to which there is a 'single critical vital system, the brain, whose irreversible destruction is both a necessary and sufficient condition in considering an individual as dead'. However, this formulation is disputed by Roelofs (1978, p. 40) who argues that the term brain death refers to a set of criteria, not a concept, since 'no description of a patient's condition can be equivalent to the statement that he is dead'. Brain death and cerebral death, he argues, 'are not new concepts or definitions of death; indeed, they are not even candidates for such roles. But although it is impossible to suppose that brain death and cerebral death can function as kinds or alternative concepts of death, it is at least initially plausible that they might function as criteria of death'. (ibid.) Against Korein's view that brain death is synonymous with the death of the individual, Roelofs maintains that, as a criterion of death, the condition described as brain death amounts to criteria for recognising that the person is dead. On these terms a diagnosis of brain death at best supports 'the judgement that a person is dead even when degenerative change is being held at bay by mechanical perfusion and ventilation'. (ibid.)

Is Brain Death a Technical Concept?

One solution to the question of whether the term brain death refers to a concept or a set of criteria is to say that it is a very special type of concept which has a specific meaning to those acquainted with recent developments in medical science. This compromise has been suggested by Walton, (1980, p. 53) who argues that brain death is a concept of death 'over and above the particular sets of diagnostic criteria that are being proposed'. But, according to Walton, it is 'more of a concept of medical science than a concept of death *simpliciter*'. (ibid.) On these terms the problem of whether brain death refers to a concept or a set of criteria, says Walton, seems to originate in the fact that the expression 'brain death' functions as 'a bridge between the concept of death and the diagnostic criteria for the determination of death'. (ibid.) Walton interprets brain death as a 'target concept' specific to medical science, which should not be strictly identified with the criteria themselves. (ibid., p. 52) The problem with this formulation is that, while it correctly recognises that the term brain death expresses a concept that has been necessitated by technological developments, it entails a suggestion that a new form of death is being proposed, the knowledge of which is exclusive to medical science. Since it will be maintained throughout this text that the concept of death is singular, that *there cannot be any sense in which there can be alternative or new ways of being dead*, it is necessary to examine the claim that brain death amounts to a new concept of death.

Is Brain Death a New Concept?

Until the 1950s the cardio-respiratory concept of death was dominant, and cessation of pulse and respiration were in themselves valid criteria for death. Since then, thousands of patients who would formerly have been pronounced dead following cardiac arrest have been resuscitated and have completely recovered. Developments in resuscitative technology, open-heart surgery and the employment of life-support machines, made the traditional concept of death outdated. Within a short time, cardio-respiratory resuscitative teams had adopted criteria for *not* resuscitating, namely when respiratory and circulatory functions have been absent for long enough to cause brain death. From then onwards it was but a short conceptual step to regard the brain, rather than the heart, as the critical system. Experience taught that between five and ten minutes of absent circulation was more than sufficient to cause the death of the brain. But the precise definition of 'long enough' was not straightforward. Such variables as body temperature and the age of the patient were of considerable importance. This might suggest that, if brain death is a new concept of death, then it was one in which criteria had become a matter of sophisticated medical judgement, whereas previously the physician merely confirmed what was obvious to everyone. But, whilst the criteria for brain death differ from traditional criteria, there is, nevertheless, considerable justification for saying that brain death does not represent a new concept of death, but rather a situation demanding that different criteria be fulfilled. This view is held by Korein (1978) who argues that brain death does not represent a new concept, but rather the application of more stringent criteria for the existing concept of death.

Can Brain Death Coexist With the Traditional Concept of Death?

Quite clearly, the concept of brain death represents a departure from the traditional concept in some respects. But does it entail a new way of being dead? Does it even make sense to speak of a new way of being dead, as opposed to a new way of dying? Objections to the very term brain death have been made, on the grounds that it could easily lead to misuse and confusion. Veatch (1978b) argues that terms like brain death should only be transitional. Either the patient is dead or he is not, in an absolute sense. Being brain dead can suggest a special way of being dead, which like 'virtually dead' is misleading.

In the light of these problems in locating the meaning of brain death it is important to formulate a definition of brain death which corresponds to ordinary concepts of death whilst, at the same time, acknowledging the inadequacy of other concepts of death. It will be maintained here that *brain death is a radical reformulation of traditional concepts of death rather than a new concept, since there is no new way of being dead*, and that it marks an improvement on cardio-respiratory formulations since under certain circumstances the latter states may be reversible. It is in this sense that the term brain death can be used as a better formulation of the concept of death. When fully articulated it is *not so much a new concept as the formulation of a definition of death where previously none existed.*

Conclusion

The concept of death is necessarily linked to an irreversible physical change in the state of the organism as a whole. Given the potential reversibility of states associated with the traditional cardio-respiratory concept, it has been argued here that only a brain-related concept can provide a necessary and sufficient basis for the death of the organism as a whole. Although brain death is an expression that has emerged in the context of recent developments in medical science, it cannot be described as an alternative form of death. However, towards the end of this chapter it was suggested that brain death is not so much a new concept but rather, when clearly articulated, it is both a definition and an explanation of death where previously none existed. That is to say, in a very important sense, the traditional cardio-respiratory concept never provided adequate criteria for death and, in the light of contemporary knowledge about the mechanics of brain death, irreversible cardio-respiratory arrest was merely an indication that brain death was imminent. In the following chapter greater precision regarding the definition of death will be sought in an examination of the three main formulations of brain death.

3 THREE FORMULATIONS OF BRAIN DEATH

> If we are aware of what indicates life, which everyone may be supposed to know, though perhaps no one can say that he truly and clearly understands what constitutes it, we have at once arrived at the discrimination of death. It is the cessation of the phenomena with which we are so especially familiar — the phenomena of life.
>
> J.G. Smith, *Principles of Forensic Medicine*, 1821.

Introduction

One of the problems in providing a suitable definition of brain death is that in the literature on the subject three distinct, but related, formulations of the concept can be discerned. The first maintains that there are two concepts of death (classical death and brain death) and alternative sets of criteria. The second formulation maintains that there is but one concept of death, which is undetermined, and two alternative sets of criteria. The third formulation stresses that there is one concept of death and only one set of relevant criteria.

Two Concepts and Two Sets of Criteria

According to the first formulation, there are two types of death. Two sets of criteria are therefore employed in medical practice. They are (1) traditional criteria based on the cessation of heart and lung function, and (2) neurological criteria to be used where sophisticated technology renders traditional criteria inappropriate. This formulation has been incorporated into a number of US statutes on brain death, and is expressed clearly in the Kansas statute, enacted in 1970:

(I) A person will be considered medically and legally dead if, in the opinion of a physician, based on ordinary standards of medical practice, there is the absence of spontaneous respiratory and cardiac function and, because of the disease or condition which caused, directly or indirectly, these functions to cease, or because of the passage of time since these functions ceased, attempts at resuscitation are considered hopeless; and, in this event, death will have occurred at the time these functions ceased; or

(II) A person will be considered medically and legally dead if, in the opinion of a physician, based on ordinary standards of medical practice, there is the absence of spontaneous brain function; and if based on ordinary standards of medical practice, during reasonable attempts to either maintain or restore spontaneous circulatory or respiratory function in the absence of aforesaid brain function, it appears that further attempts at resuscitation or supportive maintenance will not succeed, death will have occurred at the time these conditions first coincide. Death is to be pronounced before artificial means of supporting respiratory and circulatory function are terminated and before any vital organ is removed for the purposes of transplantation. (Law of March 17, 1970, ch. 378 (1970) Kan. Laws 994.)

Following Kansas, at least five states enacted statutes where brain death was referred to as an alternative definition of death. These included Maryland, who in 1972 passed an identical statute, and Virginia in 1972, New Mexico in 1973, Alaska in 1974 and Oregon in 1975. They all share the misconception that there are two types of death and the belief that there is a special and possibly premature death for organ donors, since the final sentence of the alternative definition appears to have been inspired by the need to provide a definition of death solely for organ donors. According to Ian Kennedy (1971) the Kansas statute suggests that death may occur at two distinct points during the process of dying. A patient 'X at a certain stage in the process of dying may be pronounced dead, whereas Y, having arrived at the same point, is not said to be dead'. This leads to the anomaly to which Capron and Kass (1980, p. 60) have drawn attention, namely that one can be simultaneously dead and not dead, depending on which alternative is chosen. For example, a patient may meet brain-death criteria and be declared dead under the statute's specific transplant definition. But if the potential recipient dies before transplantation has taken place and the heart and other organs are no longer required, what status does the patient then have? Do the doctors then have to use the alternative criteria based on the heart and respiratory system and if so, should the patient be subsequently rediagnosed as alive?

Suppose that Mr Smith, a dying patient in University Hospital, is found to be immunologically well-matched with Mr Jones a University Hospital patient awaiting a heart transplant. Under the special transplantation 'definition' Smith is then declared dead, but just as the surgeons are about to remove Smith's heart, Jones suddenly dies. The doctors then decide that Smith is no longer needed as an organ donor. His condition does not meet the standards for declaring death in non-donors. Is Smith 'dead' or 'alive'?

Criticism of the Kansas statute has focused on its assumption of two separate concepts of death. However, its defenders point out that it need not be interpreted as offering two alternative concepts of death. Walton, (1980, p. 10) for example, argues that 'It could be interpreted as leaving the question of the concept of death open-ended while formulating two sets of criteria for death.' Nevertheless, it is hard to see how this exonerates the Kansas statute from the charge of ambiguity. Walton's interpretation simply highlights the statute's conceptual vagueness: if the concept is open-ended, then there are no reliable conceptual guidelines from which the criteria and tests may be derived. In its present formulation the Kansas statute is ambiguous. It places an intolerable burden on physicians who have to decide which set of criteria to apply. Apart from its inherent ambiguity, legislation based on a dual concept of death can lead into a medico-legal minefield, particularly when the choice of criteria may yield conflicting times of death. This becomes acute when disputes as to the time of death may have implications for inheritance claims.

One Concept and Two Sets of Criteria

The second formulation maintains that there is one concept of death but two alternative sets of criteria. As Korein (1978, p. 20) puts it:

It should be made unmistakably clear that we are not dealing with a conceptual duality. Brain death is essential to any concept pertaining to the death of a person. What we are considering are dual criteria in deriving the diagnosis of death. That is, death may be diagnosed either by the 'classical' criteria, which relate to vital functions or, under highly circumscribed conditions, by the criteria for brain death.

In response to the anomalies inherent in the Kansas statute and subsequent legislation, a similar formulation has been offered by Capron and Kass, and others. As with Korein's definition of brain death, the Capron-Kass (1980, p. 64) proposal outlines a definition of death as a single phenomenon that can be determined by brain-related criteria, in contexts where vital functions are being artificially maintained, whilst still acknowledging the validity of traditional criteria for the vast majority of cases. Their proposal states:

> A person will be considered dead if in the announced opinion of a physician, based on ordinary standards of medical practice, he has experienced an irreversible cessation of spontaneous respiratory and circulatory functions. In the event that artificial means of support preclude a determination that these functions have ceased, a person will be considered dead if in the announced opinion of a physician, based on ordinary standards of medical practice, he has experienced an irreversible cessation of spontaneous brain functions. Death will have occurred at the time when the relevant functions ceased.

This proposal has been well-received. Walton (1980, p. 11) points out how:

> it makes it quite clear that the two criteria for determination of death are being postulated and, thus, avoids the suspicion of conceptual pluralism. In addition, it removes further uncertainties of application by specifying the circumstances under which the brain-related criteria are to be used.

The Capron-Kass proposal stresses the need for a statute which speaks of the death of a person, which concentrates on the death of the individual as a whole. This would allow for residual life in certain organs after the death of the person. It concentrates on the *single* phenomenon of death and is to be applied uniformly, not left to the unguided discretion of physicians. Unlike the Kansas statute it does not attempt to establish a special kind of death called 'brain death'. Instead it proposes 'two standards gauged by different functions, for measuring different manifestations of the same phenomenon'. (Capron and Kass, 1980, p. 65) Thus 'if cardiac and pulmonary functions have ceased, brain functions cannot continue; if there is no brain activity and respiration has to be maintained artificially, the same state (i.e. death) exists'.

The Capron-Kass proposal was adopted by Michigan and West

Virginia in 1975, and by Louisiana and Iowa in 1976, and by Montana in 1977. This legislation reflects a unitary concept of death with two sets of criteria: (1) irreversible cessation of spontaneous respiratory and circulatory function and, when this cannot be determined, (2) irreversible cessation of spontaneous brain functions.

With minor amendments the substance of this formulation was incorporated into the recommendations of the President's Commission for the Study of Ethical Problems in Medicine and Biomedical and Behavioural Research, in a volume entitled *Defining Death* (hereafter *DD*, 1981) in July 1981. The Commission proposed a Uniform Declaration of Death Act (ibid., p.2 hereafter UDDA), according to which

> an individual who has sustained either (i) irreversible cessation of circulatory and respiratory functions, or (ii) irreversible cessation of all functions of the entire brain, including the brainstem, is dead. A determination of death must be made in accordance with accepted medical standards.

This proposal is now statute law in at least eleven states.

The dualistic criteria for death inherent in the Capron-Kass proposal and the UDDA formulation, has been criticised on a number of grounds. Criticisms of the Commission's requirement for the 'irreversible cessation of all functions of the entire brain' will be considered in Chapter 5, where 'whole' and 'part' brain formulations will be contrasted. Our present concern is with the set of criteria, based on 'irreversible cessation of circulatory and respiratory functions'. According to two critics of the President's Commission's report, Culver and Gert, (1982, p. 192) this formulation is highly ambiguous, lending itself to three interpretations, none of which can be regarded as an acceptable criterion of death. It can mean either (1) irreversible cessation of *spontaneous* circulatory and respiratory functions, which is the alternative specified in the Capron-Kass proposal, or (2) irreversible cessation of *artificially supported* circulatory and respiratory functions. It might even refer to (3) a hybrid compromise referring to 'irreversible loss of both spontaneous and artificially supported circulatory and respiratory functions'. Culver and Gert point out that, the first interpretation cannot serve as a criterion of death since it would include patients receiving long-term artificial ventilation, or those fitted with pacemakers. As such, it is a necessary but not a sufficient component of the definition of death. The second interpretation, 'irreversible cessation of artificially supported circulatory and respiratory functions', does not fulfil requirements for a definition of death. This may be a sufficient condition for death but it is not a necessary one because, as the Commission acknowledges, someone whose circulation is being artificially maintained, but whose total brain functions have irreversibly ceased, is nevertheless dead. The third interpretation, which combines (1) and (2), is equally unsatisfactory since it would entail that 'irreversible loss of artificially supported circulatory and respiratory functions is a necessary condition for death'.

If, as the critics maintain, there is no acceptable interpretation of the phrase 'irreversible loss of circulatory and respiratory functions' that will provide an acceptable criterion of death, then why did the Capron-Kass proposal and the President's Commission adopt two sets of criteria for death? Why retain criteria which are based on an outmoded concept of death? The answer is to be the Commission's expressed wish to avoid appearing as advocates of radical change. This outweighed demand for theoretical consistency. In a subsection headed 'Incremental (Not Radical) Change', the Commission points out that while

> most Americans still feel that they recognise the manifest signs of death . . . [the] 'whole brain' signs of life and death are less well comprehended by non-specialists . . . The heart and lungs move when they work; the brain does not. Thus, since any incorporation of brain-oriented standards into the law necessarily changes somewhat the *type* of measures permitted, a statute will be more acceptable the less it otherwise changes legal rules. (*DD*, 1981, pp. 58-9)

The problem is that the change in the criteria for death necessitated by resuscitation technology, *does* require a radical reformation of concepts of death and human life, and that contrary to the President's Commission such a redefinition cannot be viewed as a mere supplement to the traditional concept. Such a reformulation must exclude all possibilities of reversibility which is why the traditional cardiorespiratory-based concept cannot serve as an alternative definition. However, if continuity is to be maintained, the new formulation must provide a satisfactory account of the status of the traditional definition. Moreover, the conceptual challenge initiated by brain-related criteria for death cannot be avoided by appeals to what the public may or may not immediately comprehend. In 1974 Fox and Swazey (p. 334), authors of *The Courage to Fail*, recognised that:

The introduction of the concept 'brain death' and its implications has only begun to be explored. But this at once symbolic and organic transposition of the primary site of death from the heart and lungs to the brain has already created new ambiguities about what constitutes life and humanness rather than mere existence.

Brain death is an entity produced by modern technology. The problems and ambiguities it has raised have radical implications, which must be confronted. The President's Commission recognised that mechanical ventilators and related therapy can now enable physicians to reverse the failure of respiration and circulation in cases of cardiac arrest. If blood-flow to the brain is restored quickly enough, unassisted breathing may return. However, the brain cannot regenerate neurons to replace those that have permanently stopped functioning. Hence prolonged periods without oxygen (anoxia) may lead to the complete and irreversible loss of all brain functions. Given that life is essentially a matter of organisation, the moment of death is not the cessation of breathing and circulation but when breathing and circulation lack neurological integration. Drawing from evidence presented in July 1980, the Commission (*DD*, 1981, p. 6) concluded that proof of the irreversible absence of all functions in the entire brain, including the brainstem, provides a highly reliable means for declaring death for respirator-maintained patients.

It is clear from the very nature and purpose of the Commission's report that it recognised the extent to which the advent of resuscitation technology had rendered traditional concepts and criteria theoretically and clinically anachronistic. But its concern in promoting a Uniform Declaration of Death Act was to establish legislation couched in a language devised to convey the impression that no significant change was required. This involved a compromise between politico-legal pragmatism on the one hand, and philosophical rigour and clinical accuracy on the other. This compromise is manifested in the Commission's argument that their proposed legislation should supplement rather than supplant the existing legal concept on the grounds that brain-related criteria would only be applied in a limited number of cases:

The conservative nature of the reform here proposed will be more apparent if the statute refers explicitly to the existing cardio-pulmonary standard for determination of death. The brain-based standard is, after all, merely supplementary to the older standard, which will continue to be adequate in the overwhelming majority of cases in the foreseeable future. Indeed, of all hospital deaths at four acute hospitals in the Commission's survey, only about 8 per cent could have been declared dead by neurological criteria prior to cardiac arrest. The study clearly illustrates that the use of cardio-pulmonary criteria predominates. In the first place, the brain-based criteria are relevant only to a limited patient population (i.e. comatose patients on respirators). Even among this population, only one-fourth of those who died at the four acute centres in the Com-mission's study met the brain-based criteria before meeting the cardio-pulmonary standard. (*DD*, 1981, p. 59)

In the foreseeable future, brain-related criteria will admittedly con-tinue to be confined to a limited number of cases where mechanical support is employed. But, according to the President's Commission, the 'older standard' is a *definition* of death, not a test for the *prediction* of the death of the organism as a whole. This contrasts sharply with its recognition that the 'older standard' was a test for prolonged absence of *spontaneous* circulatory and respiratory functions which, because of technological intervention, is no longer adequate. What the Commis-sion presented as an alternative standard to the brain-related definition is really a test to show that, in certain circumstances, the permanent non-functioning of the organism as a whole can be predicted.

The problem with the Commission's proposals for a Uniform Declaration of Death Act and with other proposals for dual criteria of death, is that an outmoded concept of death is promoted for legal prag-matic purposes rather than out of a desire for conformity with theor-etical and clinical requirements. It may be the case that a peasant community in the backwoods will not have access to mechanical ventilation and cardiac resuscitation facilities and that, for all practical purposes, death is inevitable with the onset of irreversible cardio-respiratory arrest. But the death of the organism as a whole does not occur, either in the backwoods or in the most expensively equipped university hospital, until the brain, the critical system, is no longer capable of integrating the vital subsystems. Anxious to avoid radical change, the Commission proposed a statutory definition of death which is theoretically inadequate. It has thereby arrived at the proposal for a statute with two independent sets of criteria for death which possesses all the flaws of previous statutes criticised in its own report.

One Concept and One Set of Criteria

The third formulation is based on the idea that there is a single concept of death, which is brain death, and that concept and criteria complement each other. Accordingly, the crucial question in deciding whether someone is dead is whether or not brain functions persist. The criteria derived from this concept must ultimately refer to the state of the brain. One must note that this formulation for the concept and criteria for death is significantly different from the Kansas statute, the Capron-Kass proposal and the formulation proposed by the President's Commission. Whilst these formulations specify alternative sets of criteria, they leave the concept of death open-ended, and the philosophic question, regarding what shall count as the death of the individual, is left undetermined. This is not the case with the third formulation, which clearly identifies the death of the individual with the death of the brain. On these terms the fate of a single organ — the brain — is held to be critical in the determination of death. This formulation was outlined in the proposals of the American Bar Association in 1974. These were approved by the House of Delegates of that organisation in 1975, which noted 'That for all legal purposes, a human body with irreversible cessation of total brain function, according to usual and customary standards of medical practice, shall be considered dead'. (De Mere and Alexander, 1975) This became the basis for legislation in California (1974) and Georgia (1975), Tennessee (1976) and Idaho (1977). Whilst such a formulation avoids the ambiguities of the Kansas statute, the Capron-Kass and the UDDA proposals, it does not give an adequate account of the revised status of the traditional concept and criteria for death. It simply ignores them and does not state whether physicians can declare death in their customary fashion, using cardio-respiratory tests for the overwhelming majority of deaths where the situation is not complicated by artificial ventilation. However, its defenders point out that the practice is to declare death only if breathing and heartbeat have ceased long enough for brain death to have occurred, thus implicitly, if not explicitly, recognising traditional criteria, (see Veith, Fein, Tendler, Veatch, Kleimon and Kalkines, 1977, p. 1748 and Walton, 1980, p. 11) To make explicit what is only implicit in this formulation it is necessary to point out that traditional criteria never adequately characterised the concept of death but were only an indirect way of determining the death of the organism as a whole. In other words, a diagnosis of death on the basis of the cessation of heart and lungs was in effect nothing more than a prediction that brain death would occur or had occurred.

(see Korein, 1978, p. 28) Given that brain death follows inevitably from the permanent cessation of heart and lungs, it can be argued that *traditional criteria simply inform us that brain death is imminent when it is not possible to apply more sophisticated tests for brain functions.* Under normal circumstances essential organs, such as the heart, lungs and brain, function so closely together that there is little point distinguishing them with regard to human death. However, as Puccetti (1976, p. 250) argues, they cannot be given equal status in the maintenance of human life:

> Strictly speaking it is not true that men die of heart attacks or drowning or lung cancer. Rather these events cause paralysis or destruction of respiratory or cardiac functions, which causes anoxia in the brain; and it is *this* which in turn causes the death of the brain and the person.

It is the failure of the heart and/or lungs that prevents oxygen from reaching the brain. Death is not death of the heart or lungs; cessation of cardio-respiratory functions is a cause, not a state, of death: 'A bullet through the heart kills within minutes, but a bullet through the upper brainstem kills instantaneously.' (ibid., p. 259)

As a critical system the brain generates, integrates and controls complex bodily activities. Permanent loss of heartbeat on these terms, is not death itself but is only an indicator of a permanent loss of brain function as a whole, which *is* death. Perhaps unknowingly, the diagnosis of death has always been brain-related:

> Throughout history, whenever a physician was called to ascertain the occurrence of death, his examination included the following important signs indicative of permanent loss of functioning of the whole brain: unresponsivity; lack of spontaneous movements including breathing; and absence of pupillary light response. Only one important sign, lack of heartbeat, was not directly indicative of whole brain destruction. But since the heartbeat stops within several minutes of apnoea, permanent absence of the vital signs is an important sign of permanent loss of whole brain functioning. Thus, in an important sense, permanent loss of whole brain functioning has always been the underlying criterion of death. (Culver and Gert, 1982, p. 187)

This does not suggest an alternative concept of death. The traditional tests of death, of heartbeat and respiration, still apply since their loss 'always quickly produce permanent loss of functioning of the whole brain'. (Bernat *et al.*, 1981, p. 392)

As in the case of permanent cardio-respiratory arrest, a diagnosis of brain death does not require the absence of all functions of the central nervous system. For example, the persistence of various functions of the spinal cord is compatible with, and in fact characteristic of, a body with a dead brain. The preservation of spinal function after brain death is well illustrated by the fact that knee-jerks may persist for a while after decapitation.

Of the three formulations of the concept and criteria for death, only the third — that there should only be one concept and one set of criteria — is theoretically sound. This formulation has the merit of avoiding the ambiguities inherent in dualistic criteria for death; it recognises that, owing to the possibility of reversibility, cardio-respiratory formulations have become anachronistic and self-contradictory. Consequently, it is unnecessary and confusing to insist on two sets of criteria for death. Nevertheless, it is important to arrive at a position which incorporates elements of the traditional criteria and their more refined application in the context of mechanical maintenance of cardio-respiratory functions. It is necessary to recognise (1) that the concept of brain death does not represent a new way of being dead; (2) that the concept of death does not lend itself to antithetical criteria, and (3) that there is only one way of being dead and that is when the brain is dead. *Tests for spontaneous cessation of cardio-respiratory functions are consequently only predictive of death. They amount to a necessary, but not sufficient, indicator of death.* Were it not for resuscitation technology these tests would be satisfactory in so far as brain death would inevitably follow irreversible cessation of cardio-respiratory functions. In this respect the context can be said to determine the criteria. In a university hospital equipped with resuscitative technology, the diagnostic tests might be neurologically based. In a farmhouse in the backwoods — where the patient would not be on a respirator — tests would be conducted to ascertain the irreversible loss of cardio-respiratory function. But in both cases death could not be said to have occurred until the organism as a whole had ceased to function, that is, until the brain was dead.

Once it is grasped that the death of the organism as a whole is determined with reference to the brain, then any reference to irreversible loss of cardio-respiratory functions should only be included as a test predicting death. For this reason Culver and Gert (1982, p. 194) have proposed the incorporation of a distinction between the criterion of death and tests for death into the UDDA statute. This distinction, which has been recognised by the Law Reform Commission of Canada, reads:

> An individual who has sustained irreversible cessation of all vital functions of the entire brain, including the brainstem, is dead.
> 1. In the absence of artificial means of cardio-pulmonary support, death (the irreversible cessation of all brain functions) can be determined by the prolonged absence of all spontaneous circulatory and respiratory functions.
> 2. In the presence of artificial means of cardio-pulmonary support, death (the irreversible cessation of all brain functions) must be determined by tests of brain function.
> In both situations, the determination of death must be made in accordance with accepted medical standards.

This proposal echoes the definition of death proposed by Bernat *et al.* (1981, p. 393) which likewise maintains that traditional criteria are actually tests for death, not an alternative definition of death:

> A person will be considered dead if in the announced opinion of a physician, based on ordinary standards of medical practice, he has experienced an irreversible cessation of all brain functions. Irreversible cessation of spontaneous respiratory and circulatory functions shall be considered sufficient proof for the irreversible cessation of brain functions in the absence of any medical evidence to the contrary. Death will have occurred at the time when brain functions have irreversibly ceased.

Both proposals have the distinct advantage of greater theoretical clarity than the formulation of the President's Commission regarding the concept and criteria for death. They have but one standard of death: 'the irreversible cessation of all functions of the entire brain, including the brainstem'. Thus formulated, tests for spontaneous circulation and ventilation are recognised simply as tests to show whether parts of the brain are continuing to function. The absence of spontaneous respiration and circulation is not a sign of death, which is determined only when the physician is satisfied that the brain has ceased to function.

Conclusion

Whilst the Culver and Gert proposal to downgrade traditional criteria to the level of a *test* for death has a theoretical advantage over the other proposals considered here, there are, however, serious unresolved problems regarding their requirements for the cessation of 'all functions of the entire brain, including the brainstem'. This formulation, which is identical to the UDDA proposal, is clumsy. If one is talking about the entire brain, it is unnecessary to make additional reference to the brainstem; the whole subsumes its parts. Moreover, it is impossible to devise tests that will demonstrate 'cessation of all functions of the entire brain', since 'there is no way of assessing such important functions as those of thalmus, basal ganglia, or cerebellum'. (Pallis, 1983a, p. 28) There is however a reason for the President's Commission and Culver and Gert's insistence upon the phrase 'including the brainstem'. This phrase is inserted to counter proposals for a definition of death based on the mere cessation of hemispheric function. This would entail criteria whereby a patient with persisting brainstem function could have been diagnosed as dead. This was unacceptable to the President's Commission and is also totally unacceptable to medical authorities in the United Kingdom.

4 THE BRAIN, THE BRAINSTEM AND THE CRITICAL SYSTEM

Civilizations can die, yet many of the component societies live on. Societies disintegrate while the individuals involved survive. Individuals die politically, legally, spiritually, or physiologically, but many of their cells continue to metabolize. Cells are destroyed, but their enzymes still function. Which of these states are we to call death?
H.K. Beecher, Round Table Conference, Geneva, 1974.

In the previous chapter it was argued that, with the availability of resuscitative technology, only a brain-related concept and criterion of death is theoretically sound, in so far as it meets the requirement of irreversibility. But a concept of brain death must also entail the concept of a critical system, the loss of which is equivalent to the death of the organism as a whole.

To seek a definition of death is necessarily asking for a definition of life. For life, in simplest terms, is that which is not dead. This is obviously tautologous, but the point is that an operational criterion of life must be included in any definition of death. At the biological level, life can be defined in terms of an organism exhibiting the characteristics of an open-system capable of interacting with the environment, but tending towards a steady state where entropy is kept to a minimum. Entropy can be defined as a state of disorganisation. Under normal conditions any decrease of entropy within the system is compensated by an increase in environmental entropy. If life can be defined as a steady state where entropy is kept to a minimum through an exchange with the environment, it is possible to comprehend a related concept of death as a failure to maintain a steady state. Thus various forms of non-life, such as crystals or stones, are closed systems which do not interact with the environment. Accordingly they can be considered neither dead nor alive. There are, however, borderline cases involving physical states which have the capacity to interact with the environment under favourable circumstances. Thus, for example, a virus may be a complex molecule which, in its crystalline state, is not alive but has the potential to become alive if its environment changes — for example, if the virus invades a host cell. A goldfish may be frozen in liquid nitrogen and would then be neither dead nor alive. But it has the potential of becoming alive once it is placed in water. These states are referred to as 'suspended animation', and clearly involve how the system functions at a given time, the nature of the environment, and the possibility of a transition from a static to a dynamic state. (See Bertalanffy, 1967; Korein, 1978, p. 23; Lamb, 1979, pp. 121-5) All living organisms have mechanisms that store and utilise information and material from the environment. The particular structures responsible for these functions are also responsible for the organism's goal-directed behaviour, that is, its future states. These features are known as 'control systems'. (Korein, 1978, p. 24) In simple organisms all essential functions are carried out by the same system. Thus in a unicellular organism, or virus, the control system will consist of the entire organism. However, more complex organisms exhibit the phenomenon of 'progressive mechanisation' (Bertalanffy, 1967, p. 69) where specific structures are responsible for related functions. Higher forms of life have developed master control systems which perform the critical role of integrating subsidiary systems. In human beings, as in other advanced life forms, the critical system is the brain. According to the concept of death formulated as 'the irreversible loss of function of the organism as a whole', the human organism is dead when its critical system is destroyed. In this respect 'death of the human organism may be equated with irreversible destruction of the critical system of that organism'. (Korein, 1978, p. 26) According to Korein, one of the essential characteristics of the critical system is its irreplaceability:

> Virtually all organisms are replaceable in man, with one exception, and that is the brain. The heart can be replaced by a pump, the kidneys by an appropriate dialysis unit, endocrine glands by hormonal replacement therapy, and so on. A limb may be artificial, but when it comes to the neuronal cells that comprise the central nervous system, an individual is born with a fixed number that do not reproduce. A neuron may grow by increasing its dendritic tree and interconnections, and the soma may support growth of a crushed axon, but if the soma is destroyed, this is an irreversible process. The brain depends on the neurons for its function, and the organism depends on the brain. If the brain is irreversibly destroyed the critical system is destroyed, and despite all other systems being maintained by any manner whatsoever, the organism as an individual functioning entity no longer exists.

Once the brain is destroyed the human organism is no longer in a state of minimum entropy production, *no matter how well other systems may be functioning by artificial means.* There are, however, a number of objections to the belief that the premise concerning the brain's irreplaceability leads to the conclusion that brain death is synonymous with the death of the individual. For example, suppose it was acknowledged that the brain is a critical and irreplaceable system yet it was not thought that any departure from traditional criteria for the diagnosis of death was necessary. Under these circumstances an individual would not be diagnosed as dead until the permanent cessation of heart and lung functions, despite mechanical support. Accordingly, the diagnosis of brain death would only indicate a moment in the process of dying where the recovery of spontaneous breathing and hence spontaneous circulation was impossible.

One reply to this objection is that all the evidence so far collected has revealed that asystole usually develops within days, if not hours, of a diagnosis of brainstem death despite mechanical support. A Danish study in 1973 of 63 patients who were ventilated following a diagnosis of brain death revealed that 29 developed asystole within 12 hours, 10 between 12 and 24 hours, 16 between 24 and 72 hours, and 8 between 72 and 211 hours. (Jørgensen, 1973) Similar observations have been made in Britain and the USA. (Pallis, 1983a) If the patient is considered alive during the period between permanent loss of brainstem function and the time his heart stops his status during this period is nebulous. According to Culver and Gert (1982, p. 186) the criterion of death would not have been met but the patient would be dead. But would he? If death is envisaged as 'the permanent loss of spontaneous or artificial cardio-respiratory functions' the patient would still be alive. On these terms Culver and Gert's defence of brain-related criteria simply begs the question that the brain death formulation is the correct concept of death. One might still maintain the cardio-respiratory concept holding that death does not occur until the development of asystole despite mechanical support. This would mean that brain-dead patients should be maintained on ventilators until all cardio-respiratory function ceased, and should be regarded as alive until then.

If a brain-related concept is to be advanced as the concept of death which trumps all others, then the foregoing objection must be met. Now the substance of this criticism of brain-related criteria for death is premised on the cardio-respiratory concept of death and the assumption that a diagnosis of brainstem death is merely prognostic. This is essentially Becker's (1982, p. 42) case for rejecting the thesis that the death of the brain is equivalent to the death of the person: 'though the loss of one vital function . . . may inevitably *bring about* death, it does not constitute death by itself'. Echoing Becker, Green and Wikler (1982, p. 54) reject the view that human death is determined by the irreversible loss of the brain function. 'Brain death', they argue, 'portends bodily death but it does not constitute it'. Consequently they reject the view that brain function is different from any other vital function, which can be replaced. To the objection that prolonged ventilation after brainstem death does not prevent asystole and eventual disintegration, (see Lamb, 1978) they reply that this is merely a technical problem that can be overcome in principle:

> The interval during which a brain-dead patient can be maintained by artificial life-supports is at present quite limited . . . but surely it could be extended, perhaps indefinitely. It is difficult to see why the brevity of the interval should have any bearing on the definition of death. There are a host of medical conditions which, given the current power of medicine, also inevitably lead to death of the system as a whole, just as renal failure did only a few years ago.

The immediate appeal of this argument lies in its reference to the patient being 'maintained on artificial life-supports', and in the underlying — although not explicitly stated — assumptions that a patient on a life-support system is alive, and that death does not occur until every system has failed despite artificial support. Of course it is never stated that such a criterion of death could only be derived from a concept of death which would identify it with the death of every cell in the body, i.e. with putrefaction — a concept which not even Green and Wikler are prepared to defend. Yet if they are not prepared explicitly to defend 'putrefaction' as a concept of death, there is little sense in their reference to the employment of 'life-support' measures following a diagnosis of brain death. If a pair of lungs were removed from a patient and ventilated in a laboratory, would Green and Wikler insist that the patient was still alive because his lungs were functioning?

The appeal to continued mechanical ventilation after brain death simply blurs the distinction between the unique and irreplaceable functions of the brain and the non-unique and replaceable functions of other vital subsystems. Lacking a viable brainstem to perform the necessary integrating functions, the 'organism as a whole' would not be functioning despite mechanical assistance.

When evidence is cited to show that, despite the most aggressive support, the adult heart stops within a week of brainstem death and that of a child within two weeks, (Ingvar, Arne, Johansson and Samuelsson, 1978) one is not marshalling empirical support for a *prediction* of death. What is being said is that a point has been reached where the various subsystems lack neurological integration and their continued (artificial) functioning only mimics integrated life. That structural disintegration follows brain death is not a contingent matter; it is a necessary consequence of the death of the critical system. The death of the brain is the point beyond which other systems cannot survive with, or without, mechanical support.

There is, however, another level of criticism which is developed by opponents of brain-related criteria for death. It can be summarised by the question: 'Why should we single out the brain as the only organ whose non-functioning determines death?' Other organs are essential for life to continue, for example, without a viable liver or skin tissue, life would be impossible. Does this not suggest a degree of arbitrariness in assigning greater significance to brain functions? The answer is no. *The centrality accorded to the brain is not due merely to its irreplaceability; it is bound up with its role as supreme regulator and co-ordinator.* Nevertheless it might be argued that this function could be artificially reproduced. For example, in some adult patients lacking brain function might it not be possible by artificial means to achieve temperature regulation, normal blood chemistry, elimination of waste products and other features of living systems? If one replies that even with extraordinary care these functions can only be sustained for a limited period, it might still be argued that this merely shows that patients with non-functioning brains are dying — not that they are dead. In such cases, the criticism goes, the respirator, drugs and other technical aids collectively substitute for the brainstem.

This argument is advanced by Green and Wikler (1982, p. 57) who, notwithstanding their recognition that the brainstem is 'the command centre which maintains systematic integration', go on to argue that the brainstem is not irreplaceable and therefore its irreversible cessation is an inadequate criterion of death:

A more careful assessment of the lower brain's role, however, does not support the conclusion that brain death constitutes the cessation of systemic functioning. The fact that the lower brain is the element in the system which keeps other elements acting as a system does not make its continued functioning essential. It is still one among many organs, and, like other organs, could conceivably be replaced by an artificial aid which performed its function. The respirators and other life-supports which maintain body functioning after lower brain death collectively constitute a sort of artificial lower brain, and development of a more perfect mechanical substitute is merely a technological problem. When the lower brain's job is performed by these substitutes, the body's life-system continues to function as a system. The non-essential character of brain death may be brought out by some mechanical analogies: the heating system of a home can continue to function even after its thermostat fails, so long as the furnace is turned on and off manually (or by a substitute machine); an airplane continues to fly even after the autopilot fails if human pilots are able to take control. The source of control is not important; what matters is whether the job is done. The artificial life-supports now in use perform the brain's work rather poorly, as shown by the rapidity with which the death of the body usually follows brain death; but not so poorly that the artificially-maintained system is no system at all.

Despite the initial attractiveness of this argument, a closer examination of the analogies with the brainstem — the thermostat of a heating system and the autopilot of an airplane — reveal its theoretical inaccuracy. In the first place, the function of the heating system of a house is fundamentally distinct from the homeostatic control of temperature in a living body. Descriptions of living systems, which maintain themselves in a steady state, cannot be reduced to the level of descriptions of cybernetic feedback systems, including thermostatic systems, which exhibit homeostatic tendencies. (Lamb, 1979) If the heating system of a house fails the worst that can happen will be that the inhabitants are exposed to the risks of burst waterpipes and physical discomfort, but the structure as a whole will remain intact. But if the loss of brainstem function results in a failure to maintain temperature control in a living organism, structural disintegration is inevitable. The centres for temperature regulation are located in the hypothalamus and control is mediated through the subjacent brainstem. It is lost when the 'organism as a whole' has ceased to function. The airplane analogy is equally spurious. The autopilot of an airplane may be replaced by a human pilot or by mechanical aids, but there is no known way in which certain functions of the brainstem can be replaced either manually or by a machine. In this context, Green and Wikler's reference to 'a sort of artificial lower brain' is wholly misleading. Apart from the inherent woolliness of this terminology — what is 'a sort of artificial lower brain'? — this argument rests on a mistaken assumption that the ventilator and other associated medical techniques actually substitute for the functions of the brainstem. But what they actually substitute for are the functions of the intercostal muscles and diaphragm, which without neuronal drive from the brainstem cannot function spontaneously: 'they cannot replace the myriad functions of the brainstem or of the rest of the brain'. (*DD*, 1981, p. 35) For example, the contrast between bodies lacking brainstem functions and patients with preserved brainstems (for instance, following serious damage confined to the cerebral hemispheres) highlights this distinction. In cases of brainstem death — even where the lungs are artificially ventilated — the pupils are fixed and there are no movements of the eyes, face, throat or limbs. The only movements observed are the chest movements produced by the respirator. On the other hand, with an intact brainstem, despite very severe damage to the cerebral hemispheres, one may find an ability to breathe, maintain temperature and blood pressure, sigh, yawn, swallow, and even respond to visual stimuli by blinking, and grimace in response to pain. In short, with loss of brainstem functions, even with the ventilator, there is no possibility of an 'organism as a whole' surviving, albeit with the aid of mechanical techniques. What remains is not an integrated organism but 'merely a group of artificial substitutes'. (*DD*, 1981, pp. 35-6, see note 4) This is not to deny that an artificial substitute can help to restore the organism as a whole to a state of unified functioning. For example, kidney dialysis or positive pressure ventilation can restore integrated functioning of the whole, just as they can replace the loss of a part. But this is fundamentally different from situations where brainstem function has itself been lost. For here the analogy is not with an artificial kidney but rather with an artificial head. The corpus of a decapitated individual without a functioning brainstem would not be alive even if its blood-circulation and body temperature could be indefinitely prolonged by artificial means. On these terms the essential characteristics of life reside in the brain. Even personal-identity theorists who base their arguments on continuity of mental states acknowledge this fact: hence the (often ludicrous) speculations about brain transplants and consequental identity changes which abound in their texts. (Parfit, 1971; Vesey, 1974) If brain death is synonymous with physiological decapitation, then brain death is the functional equivalent of systemic death of an individual. This point is graphically illustrated in Korein's (1978, pp. 27-8) suggestion that, if a dog's head is experimentally severed from its body and kept alive by mechanical aids and the same is done for the body, 'the essence of the animal's "personality" is in the head not in the corpus'.

> The head in such an experiment will eat, salivate, blink, sleep and
> respond to stimuli to which it has previously been conditioned, such
> as its name being called. If a human is quadraplegic because of a
> cervical spinal cord transection, but has a normal brain, he may be
> kept alive by a life-support system; unquestionably he is a person
> who is aware and responds appropriately to external stimuli.
> However if a person's cerebral hemispheres were destroyed by a shot-
> gun blast, with subsequent deterioration of the brainstem, the
> temporary maintenance of his body by modern scientific methods
> does not mean that a human life is being maintained. To press the
> analogy to an extreme, we may culture skin cells from a person and
> keep them growing in artificial media for months. If we stop growing
> these cultured cells, however this does not constitute the killing of
> a person, although we are destroying DNA molecules and tissues
> related to that person.

The foregoing argument constitutes the case for designating the
brain as the critical system of the human organism, and brain death as
the irreversible destruction of that system. Nothing other than the
destruction of the brain will meet the necessary and sufficient conditions for a biological definition of death. Death is a limit to integration
activity and consciousness, all of which are brain-dependent.

This, however, raises a further problem: if the death of the brain
constitutes the death of the person, then what constitutes death of the
brain? Since any system is composed of smaller systems, what is the
critical system of the critical system? The heart and lungs are no longer
regarded as the critical system and have been subordinated to the
central nervous system. But which part of the central nervous system is
so essential 'that its loss would constitute the death of the nervous
system as a whole? At this point proponents of brain-related criteria
for death have opted for three different formulations of brain death.
These can be categorised in terms of 'higher brain', 'whole brain' and
brainstem (or 'lower brain') formulations respectively. These formulations will be examined in the following chapter.

5 HIGHER BRAIN, WHOLE BRAIN, AND LOWER BRAIN FORMULATIONS

Long days and hours I've toiled with plaguey care,
Still nagging questions asks How? When? and Where?
Old Master Death is feeble grown and slow,
And even loses grip on Whether or No;
On rigid limbs I'd often feast my eyes,
And all was sham, for they would stir and rise.

Goethe, *Faust*, II.

Introduction

Several philosophers have argued that human death is signified by the death of the higher regions of the brain (the cerebrum and cortex) alone. However, the American Bar Association; the American Medical Association and the Report of the President's Commission (*DD*, 1981) have opted for a definition of brain death ('the irreversible cessation of all functions of the entire brain, including the brainstem') which insists on whole or total brain death. But the Conference of Medical Royal Colleges and Their Faculties in the United Kingdom (1976, 1979) has recommended criteria for the death of the person which are implicitly based on the death of the brainstem or lower brain. It is important, therefore, to assess the relative merits and weaknesses of formulations of death based on the higher brain, whole brain and the lower brain or brainstem.

Higher Brain Formulations

In most of the literature on brain death there are references to the higher and lower parts of the brain which are responsible for cognitive and integrative functions respectively. Nevertheless, terms like 'higher' and 'lower' do not have any precise physiological meaning and it is possible that such a sharp division is contrary to the facts; some parts of the brain may be involved in both cognitive and regulatory activity. Among neuro-scientists there is general agreement 'that such "higher brain" functions as consciousness and cognition may not be mediated strictly by the cerebral cortex; rather, they probably result from complex inter-relations between brainstem and cortex'. (*DD*, 1981, p. 15) However, for convenience and conformity with contemporary usage, the distinc-tion between higher and lower parts of the brain will be maintained throughout this chapter.

The higher brain, or cerebrum control is concerned with movement and speech. It is concerned with the *content* of consciousness (thought, memory and feeling). The lower brain, or brainstem, is responsible for generating the *capacity* for consciousness, that is activating the cerebral hemispheres. It should be clear that in the absence of brainstem function there can be no *capacity* for certain functions associated with the higher brain. The brainstem is also responsible for respiration and spontaneous vegetative functions, such as swallowing, yawning and the initiation of sleep-wake cycles. It also contributes significantly to the maintenance of blood pressure.

Those who argue that death should be equated with the loss of higher brain functions base their case on the fact that such loss strips a patient of his or her psychological capacities and attributes. It follows that arguments supporting higher brain formulations will be connected with criteria seeking to describe the minimum necessary qualities for person-hood so defined in terms of psychological abilities. The associated concept of death will be in terms of the loss of that which is essential to being an individual person. Since the loss of higher brain functions entails loss of continuous mental processes, it is argued that brain-related criteria for death may be employed to support a concept of death in terms of the loss of personal identity. However, such a concept of death would not relate in any way to the question of continuing bio-logical activity elsewhere.

Numerous objections have been made to such higher brain formula-tions. It is by no means clear whether criteria for continuous personal identity reside in either conscious activity or in the structures of the higher brain. Criteria for personal identity are much disputed by philo-sophers, theologians and lay persons and vary from culture to culture. The status of the brain in definitions of personal identity will be con-sidered later (see Chapter 8), but it must be noted that arguments based on personal identity often assume an essence, the loss of which entails loss of identity. Whether there is such an essence is far from clear and physicians *qua* physicians would be ill advised to seek such criteria.

Higher brain formulations run into difficulties with borderline cases, such as mongolism and severe dementia. Moreover, there are clinical objections to a diagnosis of the death when there is persisting lower brain function. How does one classify patients with damage to neocortical or subcortical areas who retain spontaneous respiration and circulation? The case of Karen Quinlan is significant here. Ms Quinlan retained brainstem function and (when it was adequately tested for) an ability to breathe spontaneously. Yet according to arguments based on higher brain formulations she would have been just as dead as if she had been decapitated and just as fit for burial. The courts held that her parents, acting as guardians, might authorise cessation of life-supporting treatment if a physician and a hospital ethics committee agreed that there was no 'reasonable possibility of a return to a cognitive sapient state'. (Veith, 1972, p. 1745) This decision did not alter Ms Quinlan's fate. Respiratory 'support' was withdrawn whereupon she showed that she could breathe spontaneously.

Neurologists are not certain whether the cessation of higher brain functions entails a total loss of consciousness and awareness. It is extremely difficult to prove that there is total absence of sentience when the brainstem is still functioning and some systems may still be functioning in deeper parts of the brain. Furthermore, what is meant by 'loss of cognitive faculties'? Does this expression exclude any type of perception that may be mediated by the lower part of the brain? (Walton, 1980, p. 76) Here we run the risk of stepping on to a very slippery slope. How much neocortical damage would be necessary before we could declare a patient dead? Should patients in persistent vegetative states be considered dead? Although such patients do not satisfy tests for whole brain death and *a fortiori* for brainstem death, they may have irreversibly lost all cognitive faculties. Yet no physician would diagnose death in such cases. (Pallis, 1983b)

Whilst the death of the brainstem is relatively easy to diagnose, the same cannot be said for a death conceived of in terms of the loss of higher functions. 'It is easier to test pupils than to be certain about sentience.' (Pallis, 1983b) Although seemingly straightforward a diagnosis of neocortical death is (as distinct from widespread neocortical damage) can be extremely difficult. (see Beresford, 1978, pp. 342-3) What constitutes a permanent loss of the content of consciousness requires careful definition. The problem of how to handle a patient who has lost cognition but nevertheless has intact cardio-respiratory functions often has to be faced. (ibid., p. 343) Moreover, a determination of the precise time of death in such cases (if one ever accepted that they were dead) would be even more difficult than on criteria based on the whole brain or on the brainstem. Veatch (1978b, p. 314) has stressed what appear to be insoluble problems in the determination of non-cognitive states and he concludes:

> We must come to grips with the possibility, indeed the probability, that we shall never be able to make precise physiologic measures of the irreversible loss of mental processes. In this case we shall have to follow safer-course policies of using measures to declare death only in cases in which we are convinced that some necessary physical basis for life is missing, even if that means that some dead patients will be treated as alive.

Nevertheless, a number of philosophers have argued that death should be determined by reference to the irreversible loss of all cognitive functions, regardless of the state of the lower brain. (Puccetti, 1976) This is ethically unacceptable. The vision of a still-breathing corpse in a coffin *is* morally repugnant. How, for example, does one bury such a patient? Should someone take responsibility for suffocating him or her? Or should burial take place whilst breathing continues? And what would be the outcome if a distraught family member suffocated a patient who had been vegetative for six months? Would this be murder? Or would it be unacceptable treatment of a corpse? (Lynn, 1983) As Lynn points out in her recent criticism of higher brain formulations, society cannot afford the kind of ambiguity inherent in higher brain formulations. At best these require the advocacy of benign neglect, at worst they imply active euthanasia. Between the two is a slippery slope with characteristic conceptual and moral uncertainty. As Pallis (1982b, p. 359) stresses:

> No culture has ever considered patients in the vegetative state as dead, or suitable subjects for organ donation. No physician would be authorised anywhere in the world, to use the bodies of such patients for . . . ' certain experimental or instructional purposes'. No doctor would be prepared to perform an autopsy on such a case, or to 'initiate burial procedures'.

The cognitive and effective components of consciousness may be essential for a meaningful and pleasant life, but they are not necessary and sufficient conditions for the functioning of the organism as a whole. They are not, for example, required in lower forms of life.

Several physicians have advanced what are known as 'slippery slope' objections to higher brain formulations of death. We shall examine these arguments in Chapter 10, but their relevance can be seen immediately once we recognise that, if a diagnosis of death is based on permanent loss of the content of consciousness, then this category can be extended to include a wide range of disorders that should not be considered as death, or even close to death.

> How much neocortical damage is necessary before we declare a patient dead? Surely patients in a chronic vegetative state, although not totally satisfying the tests for neocortical destruction, have permanently lost their consciousness and cognition. Then what about the somewhat less severely brain-damaged patient? (Culver and Gert, 1982, p. 183.)

The same point is made by Pallis (1983a, p. 2) in a defence of the concept of brainstem death which is articulated in the UK criteria for death:

> I am opposed to 'higher brain' formulations of death because they are the first step along a slippery slope. If one starts equating the loss of higher functions with death, then, which higher functions? Damage to one hemisphere or to both? If to one hemisphere, to the 'verbalising' dominant one, or to the 'attentive' non-dominant one? One soon starts arguing frontal versus parietal lobes.

The final objection to formulations of death based on the loss of higher brain functions draws attention to the fact that total loss of the ability to cerebrate is only one aspect of the phenomenon of death. Loss of consciousness is a necessary but not a sufficient indicator of death in so far as relatives and friends may still react to the 'presence of life' in the patient when there is persistent lower brain activity. A *Memorandum on Organ Transplantation* presented by the Executive Committee of the Netherlands Red Cross Society, Third International Congress of the Transplantation Society, 1970, argues:

> Consciousness, it is true, is an exceedingly important feature of human existence as such, but not the only one. There are in addition other factors by which we recognise in certain patients a fellow man still alive. The deceased may be 'still present' in the eyes of others, for instance because of his posture of signs of organic life. This often unexpressed 'image' of human life is part of our culture and exerts

its influence, and one cannot put it aside as non-existent. The attending physicians should seriously take into account these feelings about human life.

These commonsense intuitions about death run counter to higher brain formulations. As such, any decision to terminate treatment and to authorise burial or cremation before irreversible loss of brainstem function and consequent loss of physical integration, will run counter to death as it is normally understood. Decisions whether to maintain comatose and noncognitive states must be seen to be wholly distinct from decisions concerning the presence or absence of life.

The Whole Brain Formulation

Despite the popularity of higher brain formulations with philosophers, very few, if any, physicians are willing to accept them as criteria for human death. Support for a whole brain formulation is presented by the President's Commission. (*DD*, 1981) Anxious to avoid any radical changes in the meaning of death, the Commission opposed proposals that criteria be advanced to cover only the loss of the higher brain:

> Extending the 'definition' of death beyond those lacking *all* brain functions to include, for example, persons who have lost only cognitive functions but are still able to breathe spontaneously would radically change the meaning of death.

Such a change, it was argued, would run counter to existing religious beliefs. However, the Commission did see an affinity between traditional religious concepts and criteria for whole brain death. For example, although Jewish writings do not deal directly with brain death, some passages were deemed to support whole brain formulations. They identified the decapitated state with death, whatever might be happening to the body below the severed head. Complete cessation of all brain functions could, by analogy, be considered as 'physiological decapitation', and could accordingly be accepted as a basis for declaring death. (*DD*, 1981, p. 11) Both Catholic and Protestant theological doctrines maintain that the human essence or soul departs at the moment of death. This is not incompatible with diagnosing death on neurological grounds. For example, '[It] remains for the doctor to give a clear and precise definition of "death" and the

"moment of death" of a patient who passes away in the state of unconsciousness'. (Pope Pius XII, 1957)

Exponents of higher brain formulations have accused exponents of
whole brain formulations of inconsistency and irrationality. In a recent
criticism of the President's Commission Youngner and Bartlett (1983)
accuse it of rejecting higher brain formulations, and of endorsing the
whole brain formulation, on emotional grounds; namely, on the basis of
an emotional reluctance to treat those with spontaneous respiration and
heartbeat as corpses. The Commission is accused of equating 'an
emotional reaction to the treatment of a breathing body with the
rational determination of whether the patient is dead.' (ibid., p. 254)
'Emotional forces', argue Youngner and Bartlett, 'are also influential
partly because they are not rational.' (ibid., p. 254) Now this is a very
suspect account of an 'emotional reaction' which cannot go unchall-
enged. An emotional response, like any other response, takes place
within a context where it is perfectly acceptable to demand reasons for
it. One can then decide whether the reasons offered provide justification for the 'emotional response'. In the case in point there are very
good reasons for an emotional objection to the preparation of a still-
breathing patient for burial or organ removal. According to the canons
of contemporary practice such a course is recognised as homicide. The
reason which justifies this reaction is that, according to both the traditional and whole brain formulation of death, the patient is still alive.

Youngner and Bartlett also see an inconsistency in the way that the
President's Commission does not give any significance to chest movements, arterial pulsation and bodily warmth of patients meeting with
whole-brain-death criteria, but then goes on to cite the very persistence
of these functions as an objection to higher brain formulations. (ibid.,
p. 254) However, this inconsistency is only apparent. Having met
criteria for whole brain death, the ex-patient has no capacity for spontaneous respiration, heartbeat or temperature control. In so far as these
functions persist they are performed by the technological apparatus,
not by the patient. Once it has been shown that loss of these functions
is irreversible, there should be no problem in recognising death. This is
markedly different from the state of affairs in cases where brainstem
function persists and where spontaneous respiration, heartbeat and the
control of body temperature may continue for years if nursing attention is provided.

The preference for the whole brain formulation over higher brain
formulations is not simply based on emotional grounds, conservatism
and appeals to tradition. Its strength lies in the contrast with higher

brain formulations where diagnostic uncertainty prevails and where dubious criteria for 'personhood' are rampant. As Joanne Lynn (1983, p. 266) points out:

> At most, with no blood flow studies and with barbiturates present, confirming death of the entire brain may take a week; however, confirming irreversible absence of consciousness and cognition may take years even if one can develop an adequate definition of what consciousness and cognition are.

The Lower Brain Formulation

Whilst extensive damage to the cortex, from trauma or anoxia may not cause permanent unconsciousness there is one structure without which consciousness cannot exist. This is the ascending reticular activating system, or ARAS, which is situated in the brainstem. Strategically situated lesions in the parts of the brainstem known as the mesencephalic and pontine tegmentum produce irreversible coma. Moreover, since respiration is controlled by the brainstem, the total destruction of the brainstem will necessarily entail the permanent cessation of the body's ability to breathe, which in turn deprives the heart and cerebral hemispheres of oxygen, causing them to cease functioning. Whole brain formulations of death recognise that survival of the brainstem is incompatible with a diagnosis of the death of the person as a whole. Survival of the brainstem is needed to generate a capacity for consciousness, and a capacity to breathe. One may survive in a vegetative state with an intact brainstem, but without brainstem function asystole is inevitable despite the most heroic resuscitative measures. In the United Kingdom, the Conference of Medical Royal Colleges and Their Faculties has focused on the brainstem. Pallis (1983a) has described brainstem death as the 'physiological kernel' of brain death. Destruction of the brainstem, it is held, precludes meaningful functioning of the brain as a whole.

The brainstem's ability to generate the capacity for consciousness and cognition is often overlooked by exponents of higher brain formulations — particularly by those who have not done their physiological homework!

The explicit lower brain formulation of death, here being argued, is radically new and has not yet met with universal acceptance. Some American physicians question the reliability of brainstem testing and consequently advocate cerebral blood-flow studies (CBS) and electro-encephalography to confirm the irreversible loss of 'all functions of the entire brain'. According to the President's Commission, 'The prevailing British viewpoint on the neurological diagnosis of death is closer to a *prognostic* approach (that a point of no return has been reached in the process of dying).' (*DD*, 1981, p. 28) In contrast the American approach is presented as being 'more *diagnostic* in seeking to determine that all functions of the brain have irreversibly ceased at the time of death'. (*DD*, 1981, p. 28)

However, neurologists and neurophysiologists in the United Kingdom would reply that brainstem criteria are prognostic in relation to the heart, not in relation to the patient, who is deemed already dead when brainstem function has irreversibly ceased. Moreover, they would draw attention to the impossiblity of demonstrating 'cessation of all functions of the entire brain' which the UDDA supported by the President's Commission requires. The 'whole brain' formulation appears to believe that the functional disintegration of *all* the main intracranial systems can be demonstrated whereas the UK code, as outlined in the guidelines from the Conference of Medical Royal Colleges and Their Faculties, (1976, 1979) is more modest, but more realistic in its objectives. It only requires the documentation of the loss of certain *critical* functions ; (namely those of the brainstem) which, as a matter of fact, are the only ones that can be clinically documented in the usual clinical context. The difference between the recommendations from the President's Commission and the UK code amounts to a distinction between 'death of the whole brain' (*DD*, 1981) and 'death of the brain as a whole'. (Pallis and Prior, 1983) In so far as the brain cannot function as a whole without a functioning brainstem it follows that, once reliable criteria for loss of brainstem function have been met , the patient can be diagnosed dead. Transient residual signs of electrical activity in isolated neuronal aggregates in the higher regions of the brain do not indicate persistent functioning of the organism as a whole or even of the brain as a whole. The Commission's commitment to the 'whole brain' formulation appears to be an extra-cautious measure. But in this very caution it is seeking to achieve what cannot be achieved. There is strictly no way, in the clinical context of suspected brain death, that loss of cerebellar or thalamic function could be directly demonstrated. The caution itself may be an important defence against proposals in favour of higher brain formulations, but it has no relevance as a counter to the lower brain formulation. With an intact brainstem, as the President's Commission recognises, life may persist in the absence of higher brain functions. But with the irreversible cessation of brainstem function the continuance of integrated life is impossible. Now the President's Commission recognised the centrality of brainstem function, but the apparent clumsiness of their whole brain formulation, which refers to the whole while needlessly specifying one of its parts, is an indication of theoretical uncertainty. No argument so far produced has shown that the intentions behind the Commission's proposed UDDA would be thwarted when adequate criteria for the irreversible loss of brainstem function were met.

Conclusion

In Chapter 4 it was argued that life must be defined in terms of organisation and integration. Essential to this was a critical system which organised and integrated other vital systems and which cannot be replaced by an artefact. The location of the critical system is the brain, whose meaningful functioning depends on an intact brainstem. The aim of this chapter has been to examine various attempts to define the critical system. Three formulations had been proposed: 'higher brain' 'whole brain' and 'lower brain' respectively. I have sought to show that the higher brain formulation is inadequate since it does not require the irreversible cessation of brainstem function. The whole brain formulation meets this requirement but in doing so does not provide anything that is not covered by the lower brain formulation. In so far as the only acceptable formulation of death is one which requires a permanent non-functioning brainstem, the distinction between 'whole brain' and the 'lower brain' formulation has less significance than that between the higher and lower brain.

6 CRITERIA FOR DEATH

Who shall deliver me from the body of this death?

Romans 7:24.

Introduction

We have so far focused on the conceptual issues underlying brain-related formulations of death. The present chapter will concentrate on criteria which have been proposed in relation to the diagnosis of brain death. The first section examines the development of brain-related criteria, the second looks at the application of these criteria. In the third section theoretical objections to brain-related criteria will be examined and a reply to these objections will follow. Perhaps one of the most publicised objections to brain-related criteria for death has been that the United Kingdom guidelines for diagnosis death do not require mandatory EEG or angiographic tests. The final section of this chapter will examine the reasons for these omissions.

The Development of Criteria

Until the early 1960s, and the advent of techniques for taking over the functions of the lungs and heart, the public had shown nearly complete acceptance of medical practice regarding the diagnosis of death. This had not always been the case. Distrust of the medical profession's competence had been evident in scores of pamphlets and tracts written in the eighteenth and nineteenth centuries. (see Arnold, Zimmerman and Martin, 1968) In 1740 it was suggested by Jean-Jacques Winslow that putrefaction was the only sure sign of death. Such a proposal expressed great scepticism and ignorance concerning criteria for death and consequently reflected a total loss of public confidence in the medical profession. Nevertheless, the prestige of physicians increased during the mid-nineteenth century as health care became more scientific and professional. The employment of certain technological aids, such as the stethoscope, which enabled a more accurate detection of heartbeat and respiration, was an important factor in the growth of public confidence in medicine's ability to diagnose death. In the twentieth century scepticism has returned in some areas with regard to diagnosis of death. In what follows it will be argued that this scepticism is without foundation, and that improvements in diagnostic criteria have reached the point where public acceptance is justified.

The earliest reference in the neurological literature to a state approaching brain death was in 1902, when Harvey Cushing described a patient whose spontaneous respiration ceased as a result of an intracranial tumour, but whose heart was kept beating for 23 hours with artificial respiration. (Black, 1978, p. 395) The contemporary discussion of brain death began in a paper by two French neuro-physiologists, Mollaret and Goulon, in 1959, who described a condition of complete unresponsiveness, flaccidity, altered thermal regulation, absence of mesencephalic reflexes, lack of spontaneous respiration and progressive circulatory collapse. They called it *'coma dépassé'* (literally, 'a state beyond coma') but did not equate it with death. During the latter half of the 1950s increased use of resuscitative procedures provided the background to a Proclamation by Pope Pius XII, *The Prolongation of Life* (1958). This was a direct response to the problem of maintaining patients on life-support systems when there was no evidence of brain viability. The Pope argued (1) that the pronouncement of death was not a matter for the church, but for the physician, and (2) that there comes a time in a patient's disease where the situation is hopeless and when death should not be opposed by extraordinary means. The terms 'hopeless' and 'extraordinary' were not precisely defined, but it was clear that in certain cases there was no imperative to continue further treatment. The statement was very radical, although today some confusion in the Papal statement can be detected. From the standpoint of the whole brain concept of death, one is not prolonging life when one resorts to extraordinary means to resuscitate brain-dead patients. However, if we interpret the statement in the light of the traditional cardio-respiratory concept of death, the suggestion that death should not be opposed by extraordinary means simply refers to the continued ventilation of patients in whom all brain function has ceased.

The need for greater clarity in the definition of death and of states approaching death was given urgency by improvements in the management of patients in coma. Before such techniques as intravenous hydration, nasogastric feeding, and artificial ventilation, few survived long in a state of deep coma. Such patients either rapidly improved or died. Improved techniques of life support mean that such patients can now be kept alive longer. These improvements occurred at the same time as improvements in organ-transplantation techniques which had led to an increased demand for cadaver donors. So by 1968, an increasing rate of organ transplants provided a background to the intensification of research into the phenomenon of brain death, leading in turn to attempts to provide greater precision in the criteria for diagnosing this condition. Although the terminology was in a state of flux, the construct brain death did in fact achieve a degree of precision that allowed a pragmatic use of the term. (Korein, 1978, p. 29)

In 1968, the Report by the Ad Hoc Committee of the Harvard Medical School (hereafter Harvard Report) was a landmark in the development of brain-related criteria for death. Its requirements were fourfold: (1) absence of cerebral responsiveness; (2) absence of induced or spontaneous movement; (3) absence of spontaneous respiration — requiring the use of the respirator; (4) absence of brainstem and deep tendon reflexes. The Harvard Report also recommended the presence of a flat EEG, but acknowledged that it was not mandatory. It specified two conditions which were to be excluded: hypothermia and drug intoxication, which were capable of mimicking the state of brain death. Finally, the Report recommended tests over a period of 24 hours to reveal the persistence of the condition.

The first country to accept brain-related criteria for death was Finland. A study of patients observed following a diagnosis of brain death revealed that, despite continuous respiratory and cardio-vascular support, their hearts stopped on average 25 hours after diagnosis of brain death. The Finnish diagnostic criteria, published by the National Board of Health, on 24 March 1971, are as follows:

The patient is dead when the brain tissue is damaged to such an extent that the vital brain functions have irreversibly stopped, regardless of whether the heart is beating. The basic cause of brain death must be fully established.

(1) If the damage of the brain tissue is caused by increased intracranial pressure (contusion, haemorrhage, tumour, etc.) irreversible termination of brain function must be verified with the following tests: (a) the pupils are permanently dilated and do not respond to light (b) there is no spontaneous respiration and it cannot be restored with a respirator or other effective artificial respiration after 30 minutes to one hour (c) there are no reactions in other cranial nerves.

(2) In other cases and in cases in which doubt remains about brain death further examination (electroencephalography, cere-

bral angiography, etc.) must be carried out. Absence of electrical activity in an electroencephalogram is not, as such, a reliable sign of death in children and in cases of hypothermia and acute intoxication. (Cited by Kaste, Hillbom and Palo, 1979)

With minor variations, relating to the EEG and angiographic tests, the Finnish criteria were similar to the Harvard proposals. The Harvard criteria have proved reliable. No case has been found where the criteria have been met and asystole had failed to develop, or where brain function returned while the patient was on a ventilator. Nevetheless, a number of criticisms have been made, which indicated a need for further refinement and clarification.

One of the initial problems with the term brain death lay in its radically different meanings. On the one hand it referred to empirical criteria for diagnosing a dead brain. On the other hand it referred to the philosophical criteria for the death of the person as a whole, as reflected by the function of the brain. The Harvard Report confused these notions. It gave no reason for saying that brain death was equivalent to the death of the person.

Critics have drawn attention to the arbitrariness of the Harvard Report's 24-hour observation period. There are many individuals who may be brain dead but who do not maintain a circulation for 24 hours. Moreover, unreceptivity cannot easily be determined in an unresponsive body without consciousness. (see *DD*, 1981, p. 25) And while the Report recognised that drug and metabolic intoxication can mimic death, the need to test adequately for their presence was not made explicit or precise. Finally, the Report offered no discussion of the interaction of drugs with other factors causing the coma. (see Korein, 1978, p. 30)

Despite these criticisms, the Harvard Report provided the essential framework within which further improvements in brain-related criteria would emerge. It is now regarded essential to any diagnosis of brain death that the following rules are applied.

1. The Cause of the Coma Should be Known. A diagnosis of brain death should not be considered unless the factors contributing to the patient's coma are clear and unequivocal. Certain drugs and a low body temperature can place the neurons in 'suspended animation'. Under these conditions they may survive deprivation of oxygen or glucose for some time without sustaining irreversible damage. It follows that in a coma of unknown aetiology, extreme caution is advised to ensure that

there are no reversible components in the situation. According to the
Finnish Study (Kaste *et al.*, 1971, p. 527) 'if the code gives no instruc-
tion on how the arrest of spontaneous respiration should be verified an
anaesthetist should be consulted in all cases of suspected brain death.'
According to Kaste *et al.* (1971, p. 527) 'the greatest risk seems to be in
differentiating between intoxication and brain death'.

2. Diagnosis Should Involve More Than One Test. The assessment of the
tests of brainstem function in suspected brainstem death, is never based
on a single test. The brainstem reflexes are elicited one-by-one, thereby
systematically assessing the viability of different parts of the brainstem.
No other area is as amenable to clinical testing as the brainstem. All
testable functions of the brainstem have to be looked for — and found
absent — before the individual can be diagnosed as having a dead brainstem.

Application of Criteria and Termination of Treatment

In the UK, the decision whether to apply tests for brain-death is left to
the attendant physician. The law is not involved: a patient is dead when
doctors say he is dead. Medical practice is not however arbitrary. It is
based on 'guidelines' issued by professional bodies. These provide very
considerable moral and practical — although no legal — support. In the
USA things are different and several legislatures have passed laws facilitating brain-death diagnosis. They have done so in order to remove the
ambiguities in the definition of death to be found in *Black's Law
Dictionary* where death is defined in terms of the cessation of cardio-
respiratory functions, and to avoid exposing the physician to charges of
homicide based on criteria which wrongly assume the heart to be the
critical organ.

There are two schools of thought regarding legal directives on
brain-death criteria. One school favours case law whilst the other argues
for a legal statute. Case law has the advantage of being able to respond
to future scientific developments. But it has certain disadvantages.
First, its fluidity renders it subject to constant fluctuation and endless
appeals for further judicial action. This may be beneficial in some
branches of law but the determination of death requires something that
is beyond controversies arising out of specific issues. Secondly, there is
the objection that court decisions may relate to special circumstances,
such as transplantation; a statute which recognises the reality of brain

death in itself would avoid any confusion between criteria for death and other considerations. Thirdly, a clearly defined statute would counter the false hope that while the heart still beats there is a chance of recovery. This latter point requires emphasis. The media often reflects popular confusions of thought and expressions. References to 'giving up' and 'letting him or her go' imply that life is still present, as long as the heart is beating, despite the diagnosis of brain death. Some of this confusion originates in misleading accounts of brain-dead patients surviving on 'life-support machines'. In such cases the expression 'life support' is wholly misleading. Brain-dead ex-patients may be connected to ventilators but this does not imply that life is still present. Talk of 'giving up' in the context of brain death is both dangerous and misleading in so far as it prepares the public mind for 'giving up' in cases involving passive euthanasia. It is important that criteria for diagnosing brain death be appreciated as something totally different from criteria for passive euthanasia, and, for that reason, it is essential that rigorous distinctions will always be maintained between situations where death *has* occurred and situations where death is *allowed* to occur.

Confusion of this kind is still to be found in the report of the Finnish study, (Kaste *et al.*, 1979, p. 527) which clearly and correctly demonstrated that none of the patients was likely to recover after a diagnosis of brain death. Its terminology, however, suggested that brain-death criteria were prognostic indicators of death, rather than death itself:

> These patients died within a day, and the relatives might have been spared from further emotional distress if support had been withdrawn when the diagnosis was established. As soon as it is obvious that the patient cannot recover life-supporting measures should perhaps be withdrawn, since continued support may increase reluctance to embark on resuscitative measures generally. Moreover, the hospital's capacity to give active treatment to patients with a better prognosis is reduced, especially when only a few beds are available for intensive care.

This passage runs together 'is dead' with 'obvious that the patient cannot recover'. The authors say that the patients 'died within a day' of the diagnosis of brain death. Presumably this means that a progressive failure of other vital subsystems followed the death of the brain. But if they were brain dead then talk of eventual death creates unnecessary confusion. Taken with remarks about cost effectiveness and talk about the 'hospital's capacity to give active treatment to patients with a better prognosis', it suggests a plea for the termination of treatment before death, in short 'allowing to die'. To avoid this position it is essential that the neurological criteria for the death of a human being must be clearly enunciated. Acknowledgement of brain-related criteria for death implies that the patient 'is dead', not that he or she is 'about to die', 'certain to die' or 'won't recover'.

An example of how easy it is to confuse these categories can be seen in the criticism that the guidelines issued by The Medical Royal Colleges and Their Faculties (1979) wrongly equated 'properly tested and found certain to die' with 'dead'. (see Wainwright-Evans and Lum, 1980, p. 1022) The confusion has roots going deep into the past. A report by the American Academy of Sciences in February 1968, (which in the field is 'deep in the past') based its criteria for organ removal on 'evidence of crucial and irreversible bodily damage and imminent death'. (cited by the *British Medical Journal* (Anon., 1968, p. 762)) This implied that the heart could be removed *before* death, which in practice would be tantamount to 'medical murder'. The source of this confusion lies in an underlying concept of death still based on the functions of the heart and respiratory system, although in many cases the concept is not explicit. Clarification can only be restored with an adequately defined concept of brain death.

Objections to Brain-related Criteria

Any acceptable criterion for death must specify the loss of brain function and meet tests which demonstrate that total stoppage of the brain is irreversible. In a Status Report Veith *et al.* (1977, p. 1748) assume the irreversible loss of brain function to be synonymous with the death of the person:

> In practice death is only pronounced when the functions of circula-tion and respiration have ceased long enough to cause destruction of the brain and produce other signs of lifelessness. In these instances, cessation of circulation and respiration represent the specific criteria by which irreversible cessation of brain function is determined.

This argument is rejected by Byrne, O'Reilly and Quay (1979) who argue that 'Cessation of total brain function, whether irreversible or not, is not necessarily linked to total destruction of the brain or to the death of the person.' They also argue that the removal of organs on the basis of current brain-related criteria is morally unacceptable to most religious and ethical belief systems. (ibid., p. 1986) Their objection can be summarised as follows: first, it is argued that the concentration on the brain as the essential organ in the determination of life and death manifests a reductionism that is incompatible with the dualist mind-body distinction expressed in the major religions. Brain death, they argue, (p. 1986) reflects a strictly materialistic position which 'reduces the life of the human person to a putative organic function of the material brain'. This they hold to be incompatible with the dualist beliefs of Jews, Moslems, Hindus, Christians and others.

A simple reply to this objection would be to suggest that the major religions could all be wrong in holding dualist notions. Religious movements have been fundamentally mistaken in the past with regard to the living organism, and there is no reason why they should be regarded as immune from further errors or as the ultimate tribunal in such matters. In this case, however, it is not necessary to engage in conflict with the major religious movements. Brain-related criteria for death are only crudely reductionist if it is insisted that the person is nothing more than his brain. Obviously there is more to a person than a brain. But to say that a person will *not be* unless endowed with a brain is not to say that a person *is* his brain. A person *will not be* without a head, but we do not say that a person *is* a head. There is nothing in brain-related criteria for diagnosing death that commits one to reductionism. One might even point out that traditional criteria for death never reduced a person to his or her lungs or heart.

Byrne *et al.*'s second objection to brain-related criteria involves the distinction between 'loss of function' and 'destruction' of the brain. Loss of function, they argue, is not synonymous with destruction, and irreversible loss of function cannot therefore provide criteria for death. They define destruction in terms of damage to the neurons such that they disintegrate physically, both individually and collectively. (ibid., p. 1987) Destruction is irreversible but loss of function, they maintain is reversible in many cases:

> There is no evident contradiction in supposing the existence of permanent synaptic barriers, permanent analogs of botulinus toxin or morphine, or yet other mechanisms that would block all brain-functioning while leaving the brain's neuronal structure intact and ready for action (at least until such time as the effects of this non-function on the rest of the body might react back on the brain in a

destructive manner). Therefore there is no reason to think that cessation of function, whether reversible or irreversible, necessarily implies total or even partial destruction of the brain; still less death of the person.

This argument rests on the knowledge that other functions, once considered irreversible and final, are now known to be reversible. For example, loss of breathing was once considered irreversible. Similarly, asystole was formerly held to be equivalent to death, since loss of heart function was assumed to be irreversible. But once physicians came to see that in such cases arrest was not synonymous with destruction, cardiac resuscitation became possible. With reference to research on brain resuscitation, Byrne *et al.* suggest that it is the existence of the organism, not its functioning, that is of significance for a diagnosis of death. Non-function belongs to a different category from extinction or destruction. Irreversible cessation of function is permanent idleness, not extinction. (ibid., p. 1978) This is not to say that, without vigorous therapeutic action, destruction will not become inevitable. But with proper supportive action, they argue, there could be a considerable time lapse before the destruction of brain tissue. 'So long as we are dealing solely with cessation of function we are dealing with a living patient.' (ibid., p. 1987) Since criteria for irreversible loss of function allegedly confuse what functions with functioning (ibid., p. 1988), it is argued that the moment of death must be determined by criteria that are based on the destruction of the brain. In support of this distinction Byrne *et al.* argue that 'irreversibility' is not an empirical concept and therefore is not capable of being determined by observation. This is not to say that victims of a nuclear explosion, or a patient whose head is crushed under a heavy truck, cannot be said to be in an irreversible condition. The point is that the observed irreversibility of their condition is not primarily the irreversibility of function but the irreversible *destruction* of the brain. In cases where there is a lack of observable proof of complete destruction, Byrne *et al.* conclude that 'any declaration that a cessation of function is absolutely irreversible is a presumption, even if well-grounded, which is contingent upon the current state of medical knowledge and on the availability of adequate life-support systems in the concrete circumstances'. (ibid., p. 1988)

Byrne *et al.*'s position is that irreversibility of function is conceptually distinct from total destruction, and that as long as destruction has not occurred the possibility of reversal, however remote, should not be excluded. In the past, hypothermia and drug overdose had brought about states that were thought to be irreversible, but they are no longer held to be so. The practical corollary is that one must distinguish beween tests which indicate that the whole brain has been destroyed from tests that indicate that it soon will be, and that only if the former tests are positive should physicians declare death and authorise donors for transplantation purposes. (ibid., p. 1988) Byrne *et al.* have raised serious objections to brain-related criteria for death. We shall examine them in the following section.

Reply to Objections

If the foregoing criticisms are correct, it would mean that tests for irreversible loss of brain function are merely predictive of death and that termination of treatment under these circumstances would be passive euthanasia. However, the underlying concept of death, 'total destruction of all brain tissue' would entail tests for autolysis (self-digestion) of the brain, which no physician or legal system has ever demanded. Nevertheless, it might be argued that it is better to err on the cautious side, and that the demand for autolysis places the moment of death well beyond any point where controversy can occur. Yet despite difference in emphasis over the significance of the brainstem in a diagnosis of death, exponents of both UK and USA criteria agree that death is established when 'all functions of the brain have permanently and irreversibly ceased'. (*DD*. 1981, p. 28) But when they speak of determining functions, physicians are not concerned with the measurement of electrical and enzymatic activity in cells or groups of cells. What matters is whether this activity is significant for the integration of the organism as a whole. It is recognised that groups of cells may continue to function long after death has been diagnosed by either neurological or conventional standards. It is therefore unnecessary to conduct tests to ascertain whether the whole brain has been destroyed if it has already been demonstrated that its vital integrative functioning has permanently ceased. This is the point underlying Korein's (1978, p. 20) equation of total destruction of the brain and irreversible dysfunction of the critical system:

> Although the concept of brain death would imply the destruction of every neuron in the brain, in utilizing criteria it is sufficient to obtain evidence that the critical mass of neurons is destroyed and the remainder irreversibly dysfunctional, thus reaching a singularity

or step-function involving a state of the entire brain from which there is no return. In this sense, there is a virtual identity between destruction and irreversible dysfunction of neurons.

There are also fundamental objections to Byrne *et al.*'s suggestion that brain resuscitation is logically equivalent to heart resuscitation. According to Byrne *et al.*, just as cessation of the heartbeat was once considered irreversible until sufficient technological developments made it possible to restore it, so cessation of brain function will only remain irreversible until there are sufficient technological developments to restore the brain to its original state. However, the weakness of this analogy can be exposed once it is pointed out that loss of heart-beat can be reversed if and only if there is viable brainstem function. And while the heart-function can be replaced by either pacemaker, transplant, or even a complete artefact, the same cannot be said for the brainstem function. The idea of a brainstem transplant is both a conceptual and practical impossibility. It would require a level of expertise far beyond the reach of the most skilled surgeon, and a radical alteration of an established biological fact: the poor regenerative ability of central neurons. A brain transplant would require the artificial replacement of those mechanisms which operate the central nervous system and *all* other vital systems. With the best technology in the world this apparatus is nowhere in sight. For this reason Sir Peter Medawar (Medawar and Medawar, 1978, p. 103) has argued that 'the transplantation of brains belongs strictly to science fiction: it is not possible today, and there is no serious possibility of it becoming possible in the future'. At the current level of scientific thinking, brain transplantation does not even amount to a logical possibility since its very plausibility would entail a radical departure from accepted canons of plausibility and possibility.

Despite the fact that brain transplantation and mechanical substitutes for the brain are as far removed from the reality of contemporary science as they were when Mary Shelley wrote *Frankenstein*, the replaceability of the brain still holds a fascination for several philosophers and psychiatrists. Green and Wikler (1982, p. 57) for example, appeal to the logical possibility of a mechanical substitute for the brain and argue that the development of a more perfect mechanical substitute is merely a technological problem. But what is meant by 'merely a technological problem'? In a sense *all* problems are 'merely technological' as long as they are not expressed in self-contradictory terms. The point is that, given existing concepts of living organisms, skills, theories and resources, this is one technological problem for which no solution can be imagined in the foreseeable future. To use an expression of Wittgenstein's: if that were possible then anything could happen. We would be playing a totally different game requiring different rules and canons of plausibility. As Pallis (1980b) says: 'No technical substitute for the function of the brainstem is currently in sight. Should this ever come about our criteria – which deal explicitly with the clinical assessment of brainstem function – will need radical revision.'

Philosophers may be permitted a degree of licence in their speculations about the possibility of brain transplants and the attendant problems of personal identity, and so on. But the fact that the idea of brain transplants is not logically self-contradictory should not lead one into thinking that it is 'simply' an empirical problem. It is both a pathophysiological and a conceptual absurdity. Nevertheless, philosophers are often prone to rush in where pathologists fear to tread and see the possibility of successful brain transplants as a purely technical matter. They then confine themselves to the residual philosophical question, which they see as one of determining the continuity of personal identity. (Vesey, 1974, pp. 54-64) My criticism is not of their speculations regarding personal identity, but of their assumption that there are no serious objections to the idea of continuing human life following a severed brainstem.

What further evidence can be mustered by those seeking to show that irreversible loss of brain function is inferior to total destruction as a criterion for death? Presumably, evidence of the removal of what was once deemed an irreversible loss of function and is no longer so considered would suffice. Thus Byrne *et al*. cite research by Peter Safar (1977) as evidence of the reversal of loss of brain function. However, Safar's work does not reveal any facts which will invalidate the claim that currently accepted criteria for irreversible loss of brainstem function are genuinely equivalent to total destruction; that no recovery has ever been observed following a correct diagnosis of brainstem death. Moreover Safar (1977, p. 177) clearly accepts brain-death criteria as laid down by the Harvard Committee of 1968 as 'the most meaningful indicators of death in the human sense'. In a report on his post-1960 work Safar (ibid., p. 178) says:

As soon as criteria for brain death were established we developed at the community level (starting in 1968) an effective mechanism for brain death determination and certification and discontinuation of all life support efforts.

The accounts of successful reversals and resuscitation which are cited by Byrne *et al.*, and by Green and Wikler and other critics of brain-related criteria, refer strictly to those cases where the cerebral hemispheres had been affected, not the brainstem. Once tests have diagnosed a loss of brainstem function, and have eliminated hypothermia and drug intoxication, no patient has ever shown signs of reversal, with or without a respirator.

The irreversibility of brainstem death has been revealed in numerous studies. Ouaknine, Kosary, Braham, Czerniak and Hillel (1973) conducted a study of 30 patients diagnosed as brain dead where cardiac standstill took place between one and seven days despite resuscitative measures. In 1971 Korein and Maccario examined 20 patients who were unresponsive to painful and auditory stimuli, had no spontaneous movements or respiration; showed no response to ice-water calorics, to the intravenous administration of central nervous system stimulants, or to photic stimulation and also had isolectric electroencephalograms. Of these, 17 patients suffered irreversible cardiac arrest, within 24 hours of fulfilling these criteria, despite all efforts to maintain circulation. All 20 patients had somatic death (circulatory arrests) within 48 hours. (Korein and Maccario, 1971) That year Ibe reported that 72 out of 72 patients developed cardiac standstill within a week of a diagnosis of brain death. Becker, Robert and Nelson (1970) found a maximum time to somatic death of 50 hours for 15 patients and Plum and Posner reported on nine cardiac arrests within 50 hours, whilst a Swedish series reported 26 out of 26 cases of somatic death within 14 days of brain death. In most of these studies there were minor variations in the clinical tests, but all nevertheless demonstrated the inevitability of somatic death following brain death. In 1977 the NINCDS Collaborative Study of Cerebral Death arrived at criteria for the prediction of inevitable somatic death after brain death.

Alleged reversals of brain death prove to be without exception, cases where proper criteria for brainstem death have not been met. For example, the following case would appear to be a recovery from brain death until it is looked at critically. In the *Lancet*, 6 March 1976, there was a report on a patient 'who showed clinical signs suggesting brain death 12 hours after acute cerebral anoxia but recovered completely during the next ten days'. (Bolton, 1976) This 60-year-old asthmatic had been taking digoxin, deltacortisone, diazepam, frusemide and a theophylline-ephendrine-phenobarbitone. 'Then he took six puffs on an aerosol device containing salbutamol and then smoked a cigarette. There was no immediate effect, but six minutes later he fell unconscious and quickly became unresponsive.' (ibid.) Twelve hours later:

> There was no spontaneous respiration after stopping the respirator for one minute. The pupils were semi-dilated and fixed. The eyes were in the mid-position and unresponsive to the doll's head mano-euvre and vestibular stimulation using 200 ml ice water in each ear. All other brainstem reflexes, including corneal and gag reflexes were absent the limbs were flaccid and unresponsive to painful stimuli. (ibid.)

Within 72 hours after admission the patient was almost back to normal. All that remained was a mild mental confusion which disappeared within a week. Quite clearly, this case does not falsify brain-death criteria; rather it demonstrates the importance of the two preconditions stressed in the UK Code: 1) the need for a positive diagnosis of irreversible, structural brain damage (which the patient did not have) and 2) the need to exclude drug-intoxication as contributing to the depression of brainstem function. Two of the drugs this patient was receiving (diaze-pan and phenobarbitone) were respiratory depressants. This oft-quoted case in fact provides a standard example of how *not* to diagnose brain death.

In fact, most of the clinical signs of brain death can in isolation be mimicked. This highlights the importance of the overall clinical context, and the need to interpret the signs with care. For example: (1) Fixed pupils may be due to pre-existing ocular or neurological disease. Following cardiac arrest, if atropine has been injected during the resuscitation process, it may cause the pupils to dilate widely. The dilated pupils would then not be the result of brainstem death but of attempts at resuscitation. (2) Absence of motor activities need not, in itself, imply a loss of brainstem function if neuromuscular blockers have been given to assist artificial respiration.

The Relevance of EEG and Angiographic Evidence

Circulatory standstill is an inevitable sequel of brainstem death. Despite this fact, there has been much criticism of the concept of brainstem death, centring on the fact that EEG is not necessary to its diagnosis. Despite the popular view that a flat EEG provides an objective indicator of death, the trend in both UK and USA hospitals has been away from the employment of the EEG as a test for death. This shift itself probably reflects the (often unconscious) drift away from the concept of 'whole brain' death and towards the concept of 'brainstem' death. The Harvard Committee (1968) spoke of a flat EEG as being of 'confirmatory value' and within a year they were unanimous in their opinion that it was not essential to a diagnosis of death. In 1978 the American Neurological Association, in the report of their Committee on Irreversible Coma and Brain Death (1978, pp. 320-1) downgraded the role of EEG evidence in the determination of death from a requirement to a 'confirming indicator'.

There is a similar drift away from criteria based on cerebral blood-flow (CBF) — the absence of which over 10-15 minutes is uniformly associated with subsequent necrosis and liquefaction of the brain. (see Veith *et al.*, 1977, p. 1652) These tests, which are widely used in Scandinavian hospitals, involve what is known as angiography, a technique employing X-rays to determine whether blood is circulating through the brain. A dye is injected into the major arteries that come off the aorta and go to the brain and its progress is observed. Objections to these tests are based on the grounds that they might — in some circumstances — be deleterious to the critically ill patient. (Earl, 1974) For example, four-vessel angiography, involving complicated radiological techniques, is clearly invasive. It is often impractical and indeed dangerous if applied to the moribund — i.e. those whose condition allegedly necessitates such tests. However, greater refinements in testing CBF, including bolus techniques, have been advocated, but unfortunately they cannot assess the circulation to the brainstem. (Braunstein, Korein, Kricheff, and Lieberman, 1978)

The role of EEG and angiographic tests figured prominently in the controversy surrounding the BBC *Panorama* broadcast on Monday, 13 October 1980. The film centred on four US patients said to have been diagnosed as brain dead who had subsequently recovered. The advance publicity was most alarming. In the words of the *Radio Times* of October 11: 'transplant surgeons have got their colleagues into a fix, because they've put them under pressure to diagnose death in the potential donor sooner than they want to, perhaps sooner sometimes than it is safe to do so'. The first patient was described as being 'purple' and 'thrashing about', when pronounced dead and was apparently breathing spontaneously when seen by transplant surgeons. The second patient had muscle-relaxant apnoea and paralysis induced by muscle-relaxants; the third was a premature neonate, in whom no diagnosis of structural brain damage had been established, and the fourth had taken a massive drug overdose and had been diagnosed as dead by an ambulance driver. Nowhere were the criteria outlined by the Conference of Royal Medical Colleges and Their Faculties (1976, 1979) satisfied, or even referred to during the programme. Little, if anything, was said of the safeguards built into the British system of certifying brain death. Yet the *Panorama* Report concluded that, without mandatory EEG tests, British criteria were in some way inferior to those in use in the USA.

The effect of the programme was dramatic. Bitter recrimination followed with the BBC being held responsible for deaths caused by a decline in the number of kidney donors. An editorial in the *British Medical Journal* (1980, p. 1028) stated that: 'By the end of the year the transplant surgeons will be able to count the patients denied treatment for endstage renal failure. When, as is inevitable, patients die the BBC will have those deaths on its conscience.' The *Panorama* reporters were, stressing the relevance of the EEG, without having mentioned to which concept of death they thought it was relevant. To do justice to their irresponsibility they may not even have realized that there were several competing concepts.

As we have pointed out, the employment of the EEG in UK hospitals is not mandatory, and its employment for diagnosing death in US hospitals is decreasing. But reluctance to resort to the EEG in the UK is not based on the non-availability of the necessary equipment. This could be easily remedied by setting up regional teams of skilled physicians who could operate portable equipment. (see Poole, 1980, p. 1213) The reluctance to employ EEG-based criteria is bound up with sound philosophical wisdom and clinical experience. The identification of life with electricity is crudely reductionist and is full of practical problems, for example the high proportion of false negative and false positive indicators. Isoelectric[1] EEGs have been recorded among patients surviving cerebral anoxia, trauma, streptococcal meningitis and herpes simplex encephalitis. (Pallis and MacGillivray, 1980, p. 1086) Whereas the clinical signs of brainstem death are unambiguous to a trained doctor, the same cannot be said for EEG criteria:

> The intensive care unit is not a friendly environment for the electro-encephalographer or EEG recordist . . . Cerebral signals recorded at high gains have to compete with others generated from respirator, dialysis machine, heart-beat, ballistrocardiogram, intravenous drips,

---

1. The term 'isoelectric EEG' is a technical term meaning a linear EEG with no evidence of brain activity over $2\mu v$ between electrode pairs 10cm or more apart. (Agich, 1976, p. 98)

people walking into the ward, blood trickling into a bucket – and even from technicians wearing nylon underwear. (ibid.)

The possibilities of a tragic 'false positive' diagnosis of brain death due to over-reliance on EEG was manifest in 1976 after a survey of drugs whose presence, even in low levels, was associated with isoelectric periods. These included 'barbiturates, methaqualone, diazepam, mecloqualone, meprobamate, and trichloroethylene' (Powner, 1976, p.1123). The return of electrical activity was also noted in cases of encephalitis, metabolic encephalopathy, profound hypothermia and circulatory arrest in cardiac surgery and also after isochemical insults. (ibid.)

According to the NINCDS Collaborative Study, (1977) cardiovascular shock will give false clues which may be misleading if one relies exclusively on EEG and the absence of CBF. When the brainstem and hypothalmic centres are damaged, there may be impairment of vasometer control, which takes the form of a shock. This will depress CBF severely and cause temporary suppression of EEG activity. The same study also noted (p. 984) that the interpretation of EEG's could be complicated by technical inadequacies, and the possibility of observer error, misinterpretations, when reading the record. It questioned the validity of reports based on a single record in the diagnosis of death.

The EEG is generated by the cortex of the cerebral hemispheres, although it may be modulated by deeper structures. An EEG may help in the diagnosis of the cause of the coma (and no one in the UK would deny this) It may also help document the evolution of the coma (which can also be done clinically). But it is of no help in the diagnosis of brainstem death. A flat or isolated EEG may not be a reliable indicator of death. Patients have survived for months with isoelectric EEGs. The EEG can show activity when parts of the brain have liquified. Anencephalics can have isoelectric EEG's. Isoelectric tracings, sometimes lasting for weeks, may be seen in adults with severe brain damage but functioning brainstems. Reversible isoelectric EEGs may also be seen, as has been mentioned, in several forms of drug intoxication. As Agich, (1976, p. 98) notes: 'Even in the absence of these complicated circumstances there is still insufficient evidence to say that isoelectric EEG readings are a sure indication of cerebral death.' There is no uniform measuring technique for achieving a truly isoelectric trace and there is even doubt as to whether the achievement of such a trace is even technically possible. (Jørgensen, 1974)

Only one-tenth of UK hospitals have access to EEG facilities, but the reluctance of the Royal College to promote EEG tests as a determinant of death is based upon conviction rather than expediency. In addition to physiological considerations (the irrelevance of EEG tests in relation to the concept of brainstem death) the attitude of the Colleges may also be seen as a refusal to pass on responsibility regarding matters of life and death to a machine. Pallis and MacGillivray (1980) have described the popularity of the EEG amongst American doctors as a 'cultural addiction' lacking any scientific basis: a naive faith in the supremacy of the machine. Physicians prepared to carry out EEG tests simply to satisfy the relatives and allay public fears regarding the certainty of death would be guilty of deception. If EEG tests were ever to be made mandatory it should be because of their value, not as a public relations exercise. However, this does raise an interesting ethical point: should this deception be practised on a public addicted to machines could it be seen as a commendable means of saving the lives of organ recipients? Let us suppose that relatives of a potential donor (mistakenly) believed that only an EEG test will guarantee that the potential donor is dead and a suitable subject for organ donation. Even if all clinical criteria had been fulfilled, there would be no justification for resorting to EEGs. For what might be saved in the short term by trickery will be lost in the long term once the deception is unmasked. The *Panorama* criticism and the public disquiet it raised, suggest that the media, and to a degree the public, are dissatisfied with the exalted position of the physician. However, underlying the *Panorama* fears is a metaphysical belief in the invention of or employment of some piece of machinery or technological development that would settle, in an objective fashion, our concern over death. A meeting of the Conference of Medical Royal Colleges and Their Faculties (180, p. 1023) noted that

> the public and indeed television producers would like something more technical; some machine that would replace a doctor's knowledge, skill and experience and which would mechanically indicate brain death. This does not exist, but if such claims were ever made in the future, the profession and the Conference would be very pleased to examine them.

The irrelevance of EEG as an indicator of death lies in the fact that it does not monitor brainstem function. This is not to say that there is no place for EEG tests, but that their role is not in the confirmation of brain death but in the early stages of the 'clinical management of comatose patients to help identify those capable of survival or full recovery'.

(Prior, 1980, p. 1142)

Conclusion

The past twenty years have witnessed the development of brain-related criteria for death and the steady refinements of such criteria. There is every reason to believe that refinements will continue and that the public has nothing to fear from the adoption of a brain-related standard for the diagnosis of death. None of the theoretical objections, outlined in this chapter, need give rise to a loss of confidence in the medical profession's ability to diagnose death. According to the Harvard recommendations and the guidelines provided by the Conference of Medical Royal Colleges and Their Faculties (1976, 1979) tests for the death of the brainstem are relatively simple and fall within the expertise of competent medical staff. They require no special reliance upon the EEG or other pieces of sophisticated equipment.

7 DEATH: PROCESS OR EVENT?

> All three were silent, there was death among them, anonymous and sacred. It was not an event, it was an enveloping, yeasty substance through which Mathieu saw his cup of tea, the marble-topped table, and Ivich's delicate, malicious face.
>
> J.P. Sartre, *The Age of Reason.*

Introduction

According to a tradition supported by commonsense, the death of a human being is an event. It is normally considered, with reference to the organism, as an all-or-nothing matter: the patient is either dead or alive. Established practice demands a specific moment of death, and various legal requirements depend on it. In contrast, dying has been seen as a process that may take several days, even weeks, especially when stretched out by intensive care. Traditionally the terms 'death' and 'dying' refer to two distinct situations. Whereas death is seen as an event, dying is said to refer to a process in which various parts of the body or various organ systems deteriorate progressively at different rates. Confusion has recently been allowed to arise between death and dying because the same technology can not only be utilised to maintain heart and lung functions in some who are brain dead, and also sustain other less severely injured patients. This has led several philosophers and physicians to the view that death is a process, with no sharp boundaries, and to the belief that the pronouncement of death is a matter of convention rather than a biological fact. This argument often takes the form of appeals to as yet unknown methods of indefinitely prolonging life-sustaining functions. (Ladd, 1979)

Throughout this chapter the thesis that death is an event will be outlined and defended against sceptical theories which maintain that death is a process which is vague and undetermined. The first section will outline the distinction between clinical death and biological death. It will be argued that scepticism regarding the moment of death arises out of a failure to appreciate the forementioned distinction. In the next section legal and pragmatic grounds for regarding death as an event will be presented. These will be supported in the final section by a presentation of theoretical grounds for regarding death as an event.

Clinical Death and Biological Death

Scepticism regarding the event of death is often attributable to a failure to articulate clearly which concept of death is being employed in a given discussion or proposal. In fact, most of the confusion underlying the 'event' versus 'process' debate is generated by a failure to distinguish between clinical death — death of the organism as a whole — and biological death — death of the whole organism. Clinical death can be defined as an event which marks 'the cessation of integrative action between all organ systems of the body'. (Collins, 1980, p. 3) Conversely, life has been said to entail the integrated function of at least nine organ systems. According to Angrist: (1958, p. 2150)

> Death may be defined as the cessation of integrated life functions. Life depends on integration of the following physiological functions: ingestion, digestion, absorption, respiration, distribution (circulation), integration (nervous system and endocrines), metabolism, excretion, and egestion (elimination). Death occurs if any one of these functions is much impaired or arrested. A long period of symptoms usually precedes death whilst impairment occurs in the three first and three last listed functions.

Biological death, on the other hand, involves the irreversible loss of function of all the body's organs. This undoubtedly involves a process which continues long after the most important organs have ceased to function. One of the basic problems in contemporary medicine is that technological developments have made it possible to prolong the threatened life of certain vital organs for an indefinite period. This has given rise to uncertainty with regard to the question: Which organs are so essential that their loss is equivalent to the death of the organism as a whole? This problem can be described as 'the dilemma of death': At what moment is it right to pronounce a patient dead and without hope of reanimation to a full human life with a meaningful existence, and yet at the same time recognise that certain individual organs are biologically still functional and potentially useful for transplantation? (See Collins, 1980, p. 4)

Uncertainty regarding the moment of death gives rise to the related ethical question: When is it morally right and scientifically correct to remove organs for transplantation to sustain the life of another? The answer to this question necessitates a meaningful definition of death from which criteria can be logically derived, that can be applied at a point in time *before* the biological death of the relevant organs. Moreover, such a definition must be in accord with the ethical imperative of avoiding criteria which advance the moment of death to facilitate organ removal. Since various biological functions may persist long after the destruction of the organism as a whole, it follows that this moment should be located in relation to the loss of overall integration. This moment, we argued earlier, is when the brain as a whole no longer functions. In this respect, integration must be seen as the crucial determinant of life and death. Life is not merely the continuous functioning of organic systems, for some of them can be maintained in vitro. As Hegel once observed: 'The single members of the body are what they are only by and in relation to their unity. A hand, for example, when hewn from the body is, as Aristotle has observed, a hand in name only, not in fact.' (Hegel, 1904, Paragraph 216) Any definition of life must refer to the whole organism represented by its structured parts all functioning in an integrated way. Conversely, death represents a loss of integration which is *then* followed by the biological disintegration of the component systems. Under normal circumstances the cessation of circulation and breathing, is followed almost immediately by death of the brain. But with technological intervention the cessation of component functions can occur at widely different times. This should not create any problems for a clearly formulated brain-related concept of death. Uncertainty surrounding the concept and criteria for death has given rise to the sceptical thesis that it is meaningless to speak of death as an event. Thus Morison, appealing to an implicit concept of biological death, asks whether the stating of the moment of death is a fiction which should be abandoned in the light of more refined criteria for the diagnosis of death. Should physicians persist, asks Morison, (1977) with the notion of death as an event despite its meaninglessness for them as physicians? A similar form of scepticism is found in Phillipe Aries' study of changing attitudes towards death in the West. According to Aries: (1976, pp. 88-9)

Death has been dissected, cut to bits by a series of little steps, which make it impossible to know which step was the real death, the one in which consciousness was lost, or the one in which breathing stopped. All these little silent deaths have replaced or erased the great dramatic act of death, and no one any longer has the strength or patience to wait over a period of weeks for a moment which has lost part of its meaning.

As attractive as these remarks may appear, it will be argued that both Morison's and Aries's scepticism are ultimately unacceptable on both legal-pragmatic grounds and on requirements for theoretical accuracy. Moreover, scepticism regarding the moment of death rests on a tendency to equate biological death (cessation of function in all component systems) with clinical death (cessation of integrated function of the organism as a whole). If this is avoided the scepticism should disappear.

Legal-pragmatic Grounds for Regarding Death as an Event

It may be true that death has been robbed of some of its grandeur and meaning in the sense that in a modern hospital what Aries sees as the 'great dramatic event' is less likely to occur. But the practical need for a specific moment has not lessened despite changes in attitudes to the drama of it all. If medical evidence of the moment of death were as unreliable as the sceptics assert the legal requirement for a moment of death would nevertheless persist. In fact the courts have always insisted on a moment of death, and have often established it without resort to medical criteria. Often a jury will determine the 'time' of death to achieve a desired result in line with concepts of justice rather than medical fact. Friloux (1980, p. 33) describes the dispersal of the Estate of Rowley where the question of fact was

> which one of two persons survived the other in a simultaneous death circumstance. The jury's unbelievable finding that one survived the other by 1/500,000 of a second is a graphic example of this objective. Obviously the finding was based, not on medical facts, but on the jury's desire to allow the inheritance to go the way they felt it should go.

Examples of this kind indicate that the concept of death as an event has pragmatic value. It is certainly grounded in a tradition which contrasts death as an event with the process of dying, which can last as long as an individual's life. Thus, for example, Tolstoy's *The Death of Ivan Illich* treats Ivan's death as an event, but the process of dying occupies the whole narrative. Belief in a precise moment of death might be described as a necessary convention. Even animals, it is said, recognise death and immediately respond to the newly-dead as objects. In the face of scepticism regarding the moment of death, few legalists would disagree with Veatch's suggestion (1978a, p. 29) that 'a point must be established at which the individual is no longer treated as living'. But how does one determine this point?

When trying to time an event such as death there are two limits where no uncertainty lies. At one extreme there are no problems in recognising a putrefying body as dead. At the other extreme a mentally retarded infant is clearly alive. Yet if we advance from either extreme we encounter considerable uncertainty. Traditionally this has been resolved by reference to the function of heartbeat and respiration. The extent to which cardio-respiratory criteria coincided with concepts of death in the public mind can be seen in *Black's Law Dictionary*. Death there is defined as follows:

> *Death*: the cessation of life; the ceasing to exist; defined by physi-cians as a total stoppage of the circulation of the blood, and a cessa-tion of the animal and vital functions consequent thereon, such as respiration, pulsation, etc.

This definition has become anachronistic in an age of heart transplants and extensive use of life-support technology. However, it was upheld in the case of *Thomas* v. *Anderson* (1950) when a California District Court cited *Black's Law Dictionary* and ruled that 'death occurs precisely when life ceases and does not occur until the heart stops beating and respiration ends. Death is not a continuous event and is an event that takes place at a precise time.' (Veith *et al.*, 1977, p. 1745)

At that time there were numerous cases where the courts upheld the premise that death has not occurred until cessation of heartbeat and respiration, 'even in circumstances where the courts have noted the complete destruction of the brain'. (Veith *et al.*, 1977, p. 1745) In these cases a determination of death was sought in connection with the time of death required for testamentary documents. Obviously, the concept of death as an event was dominant, but the event in question was the cessation of the heartbeat and respiration. The advent of resuscitation technology and brain-related criteria for death necessi-tated a revision of traditional criteria. This was made obvious by a number of court decisions which involved conflicting criteria for death. In California in 1974 a particular turning-point occurred when a defence lawyer, John Cruikshank, offered as defence of his client,

Andrew D. Lyons, who had shot a man in the head, that the cause of the victim's deah was not the bullet, but the removal of the heart by the transplant surgeon, Dr Norman Shumway. Despite Cruikshank's advocacy, the jury found Lyons guilty of voluntary manslaughter. In the course of the trial, Dr Shumway (cited by Gaylin, 1974, p. 24) said:

> I'm saying anyone whose brain is dead is dead. It is the one deter-
> minant that would be universally applicable, because the brain is the
> one organ that can't be transplanted.

In the light of refinements to brain-related criteria for death it has now been largely accepted that the moment of death, in cases where ventilators are employed, should be when a responsible physician declares that criteria for brain death have been met. In an overview of the New York Academy of Science Conference on Brain Death in 1978, Stickel (1979, p. 194) concluded that 'the moment of death is the time when a responsible physician declares that death has occurred, which is when brain death is a medical certainty'. There is, then, a pressing need to establish recognition of a moment of death in a legal statute. Failure to establish hard and fast legal criteria, based on a sound definition of death, could encourage a situation where death is diagnosed on an *ad hoc* basis. Indeed, the possibility of an arbitrary approach to the diagnosis of death was implicit in Morison's suggestion (1977, p. 62) that the idea of death as an event should be discarded in favour of a point at which life had reached such a state that 'there is no longer an ethical imperative to preserve it'. But this does not constitute a standard for determining death; rather it is a proposal for allowing death to occur. When clear-cut distinctions between life and death are abandoned, there is nothing to prevent a step on a slippery slope where ethical imperatives to preserve life may cease to apply with the onset of any serious illness or permanent handicap. Moreover, without clear-cut criteria for death there would be no point at which organ removal would be free from accusations of dissecting the living.

Further problems occur when arguments that death is a process fuse with appeals to discontinue treatment based on a cost-benefit analysis of the value of residual life. Thus Morison, (1977, p. 68) having rejected the idea that death is an event, goes on to say:

> Any dying patient whose life is unduly prolonged imposes serious
> costs on those immediately around him, and, in many cases, on a

larger, less clearly defined 'society'. It seems probable that, as these complex interrelationships are increasingly recognized, society will develop procedures for sharing the necessary decisions more widely, following the examples of the committee structure now being developed to deal with the dramatic cases.

Morison has here put forward a proposal for 'allowing to die'. He has not given anything approaching an answer to the scientific problem of determining the fact of death. It may be that medical science has encountered very serious difficulties in formulating criteria for death, but the answer lies, as it does for any other scientific problem, in more research, more analysis and better science, not in scepticism and attempts to 'pass the buck' to welfare agencies and committees.

Despite the possible divergence of scientific opinion with regard to the fact of death, it is important to maintain a distinction between scientific and ethical questions. From the ethical standpoint the question may be: 'When is a person's life no longer worth preserving?' From the scientific standpoint the question is: 'When is it correct to describe this person as dead?' The first question may be raised when one is deciding whether it is permissible to discontinue treatment. The second question is asked when one is considering when to pronounce the ex-patient ready for burial. In both cases the immediate course of action may involve switching off the respirator and discontinuing treatment. But their meaning and significance are radically different. An appeal to theories of 'death as a process' must not be allowed to obscure the distinction between a patient's rights on the one hand, and the physician's duties towards the newly-deceased on the other. At stake here are questions of homicide, inheritance and civil rights. Today the courts accept brain-related criteria for death and it is acknowledged that, under carefully defined circumstances, the moment of death is the moment when brain function has irreversibly ceased.

Defence of the concept of death as an event cannot, however, rest solely on legal-pragmatic appeals to tradition. The history of science is full of developments that have overturned tradition and played havoc with practical considerations. For this reason a defence of death as an event must ultimately refer to clinical fact and theoretical accuracy.

Theoretical Grounds for Regarding Death as an Event

How much weight should be given to the thesis that death is a process rather than an event? According to Morison, (1977, p. 57) life and death is a continuum with no sharp edge between them. Thus 'dying is . . . a long-drawn-out process that begins when life itself begins and is not completed in any given organism until the last cell ceases to convert energy'. Evidently not even advanced stages of putrefaction would convince Morison (ibid., pp. 59-60) that a patient was dead, as we can see from the following example:

> There is no magic moment at which everything disappears. Death is no more a single, clearly delimited, momentary phenomenon than is infancy, adolescence, or middle age. The gradualness of the process of dying is even clearer than it was in Shakespeare's time, for we now know that various parts of the body can go on living for months after its central organization has disintegrated. Some cell lines, in fact, can be continued indefinitely.

Morison's concept of death, resting on an appeal to the total destruction of every cell, has never found acceptance in any medical community. It is unlikely that it ever will. Moreover, there are serious conceptual flaws in his argument. As Kass (1977) points out in his reply to Morison, the argument rests on a failure to recognise the distinction between 'ageing', 'dying' and 'being dead'. Morison's account of dying as a 'process that begins when life itself begins', if true, says Kass, (p. 71) 'would render dying synonymous with living'. Nevertheless, Morison's argument is persuasive and deserves attention. The claim that death is a process rests on evidence that the series of destructive and degenerative stages may occur in an organism sometimes independently of, and sometimes before, irreversible cessation of cardio-respiratory functions. These changes may involve necrosis of brain cells and cells in other vital organs, which continue throughout the major part of organic existence and continue after death has been recognised in the form of rigor mortis and putrefaction. Since vital organs do not cease functioning simultaneously, argues Morison, it is impossible to state with absolute clarity when the patient is dead. The logic of all this is to suggest that the determination of the moment of death has a degree of arbitrariness about it. Consequently, philosophers have felt obliged to put forward various ingenious attempts to demonstrate the most significant moment in the process, thus avoiding Morison's appeal to cost-benefit criteria for the termination of artificial resuscitation.

Agich (1976, pp. 100-1) offers a highly original, but ultimately problematic solution, according to which there is a distinction between 'alive bodies', 'persons' and 'corpses'. Depending on the stage in the process of disintegration, there could be alive bodies that contain persons, and alive bodies (mechanically ventilated, after a diagnosis of brain death) which do not contain persons, yet fail to meet criteria for being identified as corpses. Hence

> a corpse is a body which is not a person since it is dead, even though there are physiological grounds for saying that there is life in such a body. Similarly, a body which appears alive to clinical observation and perhaps to common sense, i.e. the body of a comatose patient, may not be alive in the sense of being the embodiment of a person.

Nevertheless, since 'the brain is the essential condition for embodiment', (ibid., p. 102) criteria for a dead brain are sufficient proof that the person is dead. 'The person is dead, because the condition necessary for life, a functioning brain, is no longer present. Thus embodied existence ends and the live-body becomes a corpse or mere body.' (ibid., p. 103) In this sense the significant moment in the process of dying is determined with reference to the point where the brain and central nervous system are irreversibly dysfunctional.

Objections to Agich's proposals have been raised with reference to the difficulties entailed in devising criteria for distinguishing between living bodies without persons, from living bodies inhabited by persons. According to Walton, (1980) Agich's account seems to involve a contradiction in postulating 'brain dead live bodies', but, as Walton (1980, p. 42) also recognises, 'we have to remember that according to the proposal, "alive" or "dead" mean something different when applied to persons than they do when applied to bodies. Thus "X is a live body" does not imply "X is a live person".' Agich's argument is thus logically consistent but its complex distinction between bodies with and without persons is extremely unlikely to provide guidelines for clinical practice. However, these complexities can be avoided if it is recognised that any residual function in particular organs or cells, following a diagnosis of brainstem death, has no more significance than the twitching of a decapitated corpse. Once it is accepted that the brain, not the heart and lungs, is the critical system, mechanical ventilation should not give rise to problems of this sort. Continued ventilation following brainstem death provides no more evidence of residual life than is found in macabre practical jokes where a corpse or skeleton is electrically manipulated to give a semblance of life.

If, as we have argued, the moment of death is defined as at the point where the overall integration of the organism's vital system is no longer possible, then it is hard to see why the legal demand for death as an event cannot be maintained. Morison's scepticism regarding the moment of death rests on a given concept of biological death — the death of all component parts. But as we have repeatedly stressed criteria for this concept can only be met by tests for total putrefaction. The only function of such a concept appears to lie in providing a form of illicit support for sceptical attitudes towards criteria aimed at ascertaining a precise moment of death. Against the argument that life persists until the last cell has ceased to function, it is necessary to point out that it is the death of the human being with which physicians and relatives are concerned not the death of component parts. As such, an appeal to death as a process cannot rest on evidence of the survival of parts or cells. No one has ever equated these with the person who is dead. In order to establish death as a process one would have to produce evidence that the organism as a whole died progressively and continuously, which is a conceptual absurdity. It may be that resuscitation techniques have made it difficult to determine the event of death. But this is a confusion produced by technology, not nature. Merely because medicine has encountered a difficulty in resolving a factual matter is no ground for the inference that a factual solution is impossible. If indeterminancy regarding the moment of death is a product of sophisticated technology this does not mean that efforts to define the event of death should be abandoned; it calls for even greater efforts to define death and produce clear-cut empirical criteria which will pinpoint this event. If technology has blurred the traditional distinction between a man alive and a man dead then there is an urgent and pressing reason to restore clarity. To fail to do so is to run the horrendous risk of declaring a man dead when he is still alive. This is the practical consequence of scepticism. In any given philosophical context the question 'Is he dead?' is still, and always will be, a factual matter.

It is sometimes argued that a diagnosis of human death in terms of brain-related criteria constitutes an arbitrary decision regarding the significant moment in the process of dying, since artificial supports may enable certain vital functions to continue. As we have seen this argument rests on confusion between clinical death and biological death, with the resulting sceptical conclusion regarding the moment of death. The following argument by Alister Browne (1983, p. 30) is representative of the sceptical thesis that death cannot be determined as a biological fact:

Judgements of death seem to be cold, hard, scientific facts. That, no doubt, is why they are easier to accept than their alternative, the making of fallible value-judgements about the worth of lives. But it is not a biological fact that one who has suffered whole-brain death is dead. One can say that it is a biological fact that if such a person is not on a respirator — if blood is not circulating, food metabolizing, wastes being eliminated, etc., — then that person is dead. But if he is on a respirator, and these processes are occurring — albeit artificially supported — then, while one may want to say the person is dead, one cannot claim this to be a *biological* fact.

This argument is subsequently reinforced by the statement that there are no significant boundaries between cerebral death (loss of hemispheric function) and 'whole brain' death.

But if one cannot argue that there is a relevant difference between spontaneous and artificially supported respiration and heartbeat, then any behaviour deemed appropriate at the time of whole-brain death will also be appropriate at the time of cerebral death. (ibid., p. 31)

The answer should be straightforward. Criteria for the 'death of the brain as a whole' can be established with precision once it is recognised that the irreversible loss of brainstem function, the critical system, is the point at which death can be objectively determined. Moreover, a clear-cut distinction between death of the brain as a whole (brainstem death) and cerebral death (the vegetative state) is not difficult. (see Pallis, 1983a, 1983b)

A definition which recognises that death is an event must be separated from much of the nonsense that has been employed to support it. Morison is correct, when he warns that there are serious pitfalls in speaking of death as an event, if the event in question is departure of some vital substance or 'entelechy'. When it is postulated that one vital 'thing' is lacking in a corpse that is possessed by a living being, we run the risk of committing the fallacy of misplaced concreteness. This was one of the misleading assumptions of vitalism — the belief in a substance corresponding to the word 'life'. Consequently it was thought that there must be some specific thing common to all living matter. Thus hypothetical entities were postulated, such as 'anima' or 'entelechy', that were possessed by living things. This inevitably yielded absurdities such as 'to be animate you need to possess anima'. Once a concept has been reified it is but a short step towards speaking of its arrival and departure as one would of the arrival and departure of a train. Thus nonsensical locutions such as 'If life goes then you will die' become enshrined in commonsense. We speak of 'hanging on to life by a thread' or 'letting his life slip away', thereby lending support to the reification of the concept. Just as life is reified into a substance, so death is considered in equally concrete terms. Hence references to the 'jaws of death' and the 'arms of death' which suggest that death is something we fall into. Death is even given a degree of autonomy: 'Who will it claim next?' 'Death struck in the afternoon,' He has an appointment with death'. In these cases death is personified as a grim reaper who cannot be cheated. Of course these are metaphors whose role is primarily aesthetic but, as the history of vitalism shows, such metaphors have a profound influence on scientific understanding.

Notwithstanding the fact that certain concepts of death as an event rest on misleading metaphors, there is sufficient clinical evidence to indicate the moment when irreversible cessation of brainstem function is certain. Developments in resuscitation technology have made it difficult to locate the precise moment of death in terms of traditional cardio-respiratory criteria, but clearly defined criteria for brain death draw attention to an empirically determinable moment which marks the end of the process of dying.

Conclusion

Scepticism regarding the moment of death has policy consequences which run counter to pressing medical, social, legal and religious needs, such as making decisions regarding the withdrawal of ventilation, announcing burial and mourning times, interpreting of wills, etc. As long as social agencies require a moment of death then this moment should be determined with reference to biological criteria. There are significant events which indicate the beginning, the point of no return, and the end of the process of dying. As such, a definition stipulating that death occurs at a specific time is preferable to one which makes a vague reference to this process of dying. If it were the case that death is a process then, as Culver and Gert (1982, p. 180) point out, it either starts when the person is clearly alive, which confuses the 'process of death' with the 'process of dying', or the process of death starts when the person is no longer alive, which confuses death with the process of disintegration. If we regard death as a process, then either (i) the process starts when the person is still living, which confuses the process of death with the process of dying, for we all regard someone who is dying as not yet dead, or (ii) the process of death starts when the person is no longer alive, which confuses the process of death with the process of disintegration. But there is a process of dying and there is a process of disintegration, and death is the event which indicates the moment when the process of dying ceases and the process of disintegration begins. This moment, we have argued, is the moment when the brain as a whole ceases to function, when the brainstem, its critical system, has become irreversibly dysfunctional. Medicine must formulate criteria which enable this moment of death to be precisely determined.

8 BRAIN DEATH AND PERSONAL IDENTITY

> She was dead. Her consciousness was destroyed. But not her life . . .
> that delicate life had merely stopped, it floated, filled with unechoed
> cries and ineffective hopes with sombre splendours, antiquated faces
> and perfumes, it floated at the outer edge of the world, between
> parentheses, unforgettable and self-subsistent, more indestructible
> than a mineral, and nothing could prevent it from having *been*, it
> had just undergone its ultimate metamorphosis. 'A life', thought
> Mathieu, 'is formed from the future just as bodies are compounded
> from the void'.
>
> J.P. Sartre, *The Age of Reason.*

Introduction

This chapter will examine various *philosophical* accounts of personal
identity in the context of brain-related criteria for diagnosing death. It
will be argued that only a brainstem concept of death provides satisfactory criteria for the death of a *human being*. This is a biological
concept. Expressions like 'death of a person' or 'loss of personal
identity', which appear in philosophical literature and sometimes are
given a psychological significance, are unsatisfactory candidates for a
definition of death. In what follows, the death of a human being, so
defined as the 'irreversible loss of function of the organism as a whole',
will be defended against various attempts to equate death with loss of
personal identity.

Death of a Human Being and Loss of Personal Identity

The concept of a living human being' involves a distinction between a
person whose organs are controlled by the central nervous system and a
corpse where this control is lacking and the organs are in a process of
disintegration. Without a functioning brainstem the body is merely a
mass of inert matter in which entropy increases as residual functions
decline and organs decay. At this stage, certain residual functions such
as continued growth of hair and so on, do not confer an iota of human

life or personality. When the brainstem is dead, neither the human body nor the person exists in any meaningful sense. Although heart and respiratory-system criteria have been generally supplanted by brain-related criteria, it has been recognised that the absence of heartbeat or pulse were never considered the sole significant factor in ascertaining death in early religious beliefs. (see Veith *et al.*, 1977, p. 1653) Thus, in an important sense, brain death has always been an implicit, although unformulated, concept of the death of the human being. In earlier societies the twitching of a lizard's tail or the death throes of a decapitated man were never considered as examples of residual human life, but simply as manifestations of cellular life — recognised as events that persisted after the death of the organism as a whole. (ibid.) In this respect brainstem death must be seen as the physiological equivalent of anatomical decapitation which in both early and contemporary sources clearly signified the death of the organism as a whole. The brainstem concept of death implies that irreversible loss of function of the brain as a whole, not merely its hemisphere regions, is essential to the death of a human being. At this point it can be safely inferred that the person is dead. Although many characteristics associated with personality, such as consciousness, cognition and speech, may cease before cessation of brainstem function, their loss does not provide necessary and sufficient conditions for death. Like what is seen in advanced dementia these losses are simply manifestations of the diseased state of the person. Certainty regarding the death of the human being can be obtained if and only if the brainstem is dead, for only this relates to a concept of death so defined as the permanent loss of function of the organism as a whole.

It has been argued that a diagnosis of death of the person could be linked to criteria for loss of certain characteristics (such as memory and behavioural patterns) associated with psychological aspects of human life. According to this view, if the cortex is totally destroyed, the patient has lost his or her personal identity. Nowadays resuscitative technology can assist such patients to maintain life at a steady, even if in a permanently vegetative, state. The question posed by personal-identity theorists of death is whether we should regard loss of personality in these contexts as being equivalent to the death of the human being. According to the concept of brainstem death, so defined as the irreversible loss of function of the organism as a whole, the loss of psychological attributes is a necessary but not a sufficient condition of death. Psychological aspects may be absent but human life may continue as long as integrated functioning persists.

At this point an advocate of the personal-identity concept of death may object that too much is being required. If psychological features are lost, it might be argued, then the patient cannot suffer any harm if treatment is terminated and events allowed to follow their natural course. According to Agich: (1976, p. 103) 'If no person is present, i.e. if the essential condition for the embodiment of higher level functions of mind is permanently absent, then no harm or injury can be inflicted upon the patient as a person.' Here the 'person' is visualised with reference to 'higher level functions of mind'. These functions are notoriously difficult to define and 'appropriate criteria' lacks diagnostic certainty. This uncertainty can only be avoided by accepting the proposal that the point where loss of personhood is certain is when the brain as a whole, and hence the organism as a whole, no longer functions. That moment is when the brainstem dies.

There is, nevertheless, considerable support for arguments which base criteria for death on loss of psychological attributes. In so far as Green and Wikler endorse brain-related criteria for death their yardstick is death of the person. They see this as determined by loss of hemispheric functions. Residual life in the body, they argue, has little significance if psychological life has effectively ceased: a person ceases to exist when the causal processes that normally underlie that person's continuity are destroyed. On these terms, they argue, brain-death criteria do not define the death of the organism, but may provide guidelines for allowing the death of the organism to occur. Hence a brain-death statute, they argue, need not be based on a definition of death of the organism as a whole, but could provide grounds for the suspension of treatment, and hence, 'letting die' patients in vegetative or various anencephalic states. Objections that this might lead to the termination of treatment for the mentally ill, the senile and others, are met by the proposal to limit the licensing of 'letting die by brain death statute' to the 'permanently comatose and no one else'. (Green and Wikler, 1982, p. 74)

The problem with this proposal is that it rests on a controversial theory of what it is for a person to cease to exist. Personal-identity theories of death are unacceptable to British physicians, and the Report of the President's Commission (*DD*, 1981) rejects them for reasons that are worth enumerating. These are (1) Despite much philosophical scholarship over centuries, the problem of personal identity remains unresolved. The abstract terminology of personal-identity theory renders it less useful for public policy than biologically based concepts of death of the organism as a whole. (2) The practical application of personal-identity theories would give rise to many borderline problems. Senile or retarded patients might fail to meet criteria for personhood. Yet any argument which classified such individuals as dead would not meet with either medical or public acceptance. (3) As the Karen Quinlan case has amply demonstrated, patients in whom the neocortex and subcortical areas have borne the brunt of the damage may retain or regain spontaneous respiration. Yet the implications of the personal-identity argument would be that Karen Quinlan, who retained brain-stem function and continued to breathe spontaneously, was a corpse and fit for burial. (4) Diagnosis in cases of lost personal identity is fraught with difficulties. It is nothing like as easy as the diagnosis of the death of the organism as a whole. According to the President's Commission: (*DD*, 1981, p. 40)

> It is not known which portions of the brain are responsible for cognition and consciousness; what little is known points to substantial interconnections among the brainstem, subcortical structures and the neocortex. Thus the 'higher brain' may well exist only as a metaphorical concept, not in reality. Second, even when the sites of certain aspects of consciousness can be found, their cessation often cannot be assessed with the certainty that would be required in applying a statutory definition.

Unlike the biologically based concept of death as a loss of function of the organism as a whole, the concept of loss of personal identity is of philosophical and psychological origin and lacks clear empirical criteria. It is defined in terms of certain kinds of abilities and qualities of awareness. As Culver and Gert (1982, p. 183) point out, 'it is inherently vague'.

The concept of a person belongs to a different logical space to that of living human beings. In some cases personal identity may transcend the spatio-temporal existence of bodies. Thus in an important sense the kinds of things we can attribute to persons cannot be said about the organism as a whole. Thus harm and injury to persons can be independent of harm and injury done to their bodies. A person can be an object of misfortune, betrayal and ridicule, long after the termination of his or her bodily existence. Cromwell was humiliated and disgraced when his body was gibbeted at Tyburn long after putrefaction had set in. The benefits and harms that may befall a person are not necessarily dependent upon that person's experiential state. This is largely because personhood is bound up with moral predicates which transcend those which can be attributed to physical states. If, then, a person can be harmed long after the point where the harm can be experienced, it would appear that, contrary to Agich and others, there is no point at which a person cannot be harmed. Consequently, this harm could be inflicted in cases where the organs of the deceased have been removed without prior consent, or if life-sustaining therapy was discontinued before the death of the brain as a whole — even if the patient was deemed to be incapable of experiencing the effects. In such cases, the patient's inability to experience harm does not justify its infliction.

Life refers to the biological processes which maintain the human being. In this respect the term 'death', when applied to persons, has only a metaphorical meaning. In a literal sense it is human beings that die; *personal identity may in some sense survive death and in some senses it may be said to be lost prior to the death of the human being.* In the biological sense, however, the concept of death only applies to organisms. As Culver and Gert (1982, p. 183) argue:

> Thus in a literal sense, death can be applied directly only to bio-
> logical organisms and not to persons. We do not object to the phrase
> 'death of a person', but the phrase in common usage actually means
> the death of the organism which was the person.

Philosophers who speak of the death of the person, whilst the organism as a whole survives, appeal to nothing more than an abstract metaphor. Loss of personhood is hard to define and is bound up with factors as diverse as the moral stature of the person, the surrounding culture and the relationship between the observer and the person in question. In this respect, despite Culver's and Gert's excellent argument against a psychologically based definition of death, their own account (1982, p. 183) of loss of personhood —as the absence of psychological capac- ities, such as consciousness and cognition — is open to criticism: 'We are immediately aware of the loss of personhood in these patients and are repulsed by the idea of continuing to treat them as if they were persons.' This is highly questionable. There is no necessary reason why loss of consciousness or cognition should be perceived as loss of person- hood. (The last years of Churchill's (or Lenin's) life, in which their mental capacities were probably impaired, detracts nothing from their historical 'personhoods'.) The idea of still accepting them as persons is not inherently repulsive. They can be objects of the same devotion or hatred as normal human beings, even if they cannot respond like other human beings. Opposition to brain-related criteria for the death of a human being sometimes relies upon speculations regarding either brain transplants or artificial brains. It is hypothesised that these might perpetuate personal identity after the cessation of natural brain activity. On these terms, personhood would persist, and the residual philosophical problem would be whether it was the *same* personal identity which persisted. In a dialogue on personal identity Vesey and Parfit (1974, p. 58) consider the following possibility:

> When I die in a normal way, scientists are going to map the states of all the cells in my brain and after a few months they will have constructed a perfect duplicate of me out of organic matter. And this duplicate will wake up fully psychologically continuous with me, seeming to remember my life with my character, etc.

They describe this as a 'secular vision of the Resurrection'. But if it were to happen, it would entail the same degree of the miraculous as the traditional version. Unless it can be shown that a viable brainstem persists throughout these changes, then no credence can be given to speculations about psychological continuity in residual life. If we are talking about genuine resurrection, religious or secular — whatever the latter might mean — then we have moved into that spurious arena of logical possibility where almost anything can be said, providing it is not self-contradictory, even if none of it can happen.

Philosophers who have to resort to science fiction usually have an unstable case. Science fiction examples emphasise the transitional nature of personal identity to the point where it readily destroys our present conceptions. This may be a useful task. The ordinary or everyday conceptions of personal identity may be ill-founded, or in need of clarification. They are certainly not, and should not, be regarded as self-justified. But they are the only notions available and examples drawn from science fiction which radically depart from them offer little help in dealing with the very real and fundamental problems of self.

So far the minimum characteristics required for human life have been outlined. It has been concluded that a human being requires a functioning brainstem, capable of integrating all organ systems. However, criteria for the 'death of a human being' must be distinguished from criteria for the loss of 'personal identity.' Confusion between these categories has produced much nonsense in philosophical discussions concerning criteria for death. The properties associated with personal identity are those concerned with purposive action, affective qualities, and moral qualities and active intelligence. Quite obviously these qualities cannot be observed in patients with a non-functioning cortex. But they do not have to be observed in order to conclude that he or she is alive.

The attributes associated with personal identity are logically distinct from characteristics associated with living persons. Individuals may die, the human being may no longer be a human being, but aspects of their personality, their identity, may survive their bodies. We can see this in the distinction between 'being dead' and 'being deceased'. Whilst things, like engines, batteries or planets, may be dead, only persons can be deceased. This is because there is a sense in which a deceased person may be absent, but that very absence be present. Thus to say that a person is deceased is to refer to the persistence of personal identity beyond the stage of physical disintegration: 'being deceased means being absent in such a way that one's absence can still be present, even though the absence that constitutes one's death may itself be absent'. (Johnstone, 1978, p. 14) *While personal identity may, in some senses, survive physical destruction, personal life clearly does not.* Death involves a sharp contrast in attitudes and reactions towards the body that once manifested human life. One cannot feel pity for a body, as one can for the person that once inhabited it.

There are, however, further distinctions between criteria for personal identity and the continuance of life. Criteria for personal identity, unlike criteria for life, can be based on either fictional or real concepts of bodily image and organic continuity. Whilst the continuous function of the brain as a whole is a necessary and sufficient condition for human life, there can be no clear-cut guidelines for the loss of personal identity. Criteria for personal identity might be based on psychological or spiritual qualities or morally relevant characteristics. Whilst brain-related criteria for the death of the human being have replaced cardiac or respiratory criteria, loss of personal identity is still conceived of by many people in terms of the loss of heart-function. Thus for many the heart is still regarded as the essential organ with regard to personal identity. The heart is symbolic of love, loyalty and strong emotions. People speak of 'heart-breaking' experiences, and being 'all heart' or 'big-hearted' as a commendable moral attribute. Phrases like 'my heart is not in it' depict feelings about our work. The meaning of 'I left my heart in San Francisco' could never be replaced by references to kidneys, lungs, brains or other organs essential to a living person. That the heart is associated, rightly or wrongly, with personality is a fact which cannot be ignored.

In a study of psychiatric complications following heart transplants

Lunde (1969, p. 372) notes how:

> Some patients have felt that by receiving the heart of another person they might take on some of the personality characteristics of the donor. One man literally decided that the day of his transplant was his new birthday, which he planned to celebrate from then on. He felt that he had been born again and was twenty years old. This was a forty-two-year-old man who had received the heart of a twenty-year-old.

Another patient claimed that it made him feel good to receive the heart of a prominent local citizen renowned for his good work, and consequently the patient 'felt an obligation to live up to the standards set by the man whose heart he had received'. (ibid., p. 373)

Sometimes (ibid., p. 373) the family of the donor may establish an intense emotional relationship with the recipient of their relative's heart.

> In one case, the spouse of the donor called the hospital regularly to inquire how the recipient was doing, and when the patient finally died the family seemed to experience a delayed grief reaction. The death of the heart seemed to finalize the death of the donor for the family.

As these example show, personal identity need not depend upon biologically relevant facts, but on a 'body image'. Which part of the body is most relevant appears to be a matter of contingency, affected by custom and tradition, rather than by clinical evidence.

Opponents of brain-related criteria for the death of the living person sometimes point out that the person cannot be reduced to the components of the brain. But, once the distinction between criteria for the death of a person and criteria for loss of personal identity is appreciated, this opposition is dissolved. One can attribute personal identity to a being in *any* physical state, ranging from senility, irreversible coma, to skeletal remains or even ghostly manifestations. Criteria for a living person, however, require as a minimum the continuous integration of the organism as a whole. This is met by a brainstem definition of death.

Insistence upon the *integrative* function of the brainstem in any account of the death of the person avoids any accusation of a dualism between brain and body, which illicitly favours the brain. This objection can be seen in Hans Jonas's awareness that a new formulation of soul-body dualism sometimes lurks behind brain-related definitions of death. On these terms it would appear that the brain represents the person or soul, and the body its extension or tool. 'Thus when the brain dies, it is as when the soul departed: what is left are "mortal remains".' (Jonas, 1974, p. 139) Against this Jonas rightly points out that the body is equally important.

> But it is no less an exaggeration of the cerebral aspect as it was of the conscious soul, to deny the extracerebral body its essential share in the identity of the person. The body is as uniquely the body of this brain and no other, as the brain is uniquely the brain of this body and no other. What is under the brain's central control, the bodily total, is as individual, as much 'myself', as singular to my identity (fingerprints!), as noninterchangeable, as the controlling (and reciprocally controlled) brain itself. My identity is the identity of the whole organism, even if the higher functions of personhood are seated in the brain. How else could a man love a woman and not merely her brains? How else could we lose ourselves in the aspect of a face? Be touched by the delicacy of a frame? It's this person's, and no one elses. Therefore, the body of the comatose, as long as — even with the help of art — it still breathes, pulses, and functions otherwise, must still be considered a residual continuance of the subject that loved and was loved, and as such is still entitled to some of the sacrosanctity accorded to such a subject by the laws of God and men.

Jonas is correct in so far as his remarks are directed against higher brain formulations, which see death as the loss of certain characteristics associated with personal identity while the continuing function of the brainstem maintains the integration of the organism as a whole. Human life depends on more than continuing function of the cerebral hemispheres. But, according to the brainstem definition, death does not occur until both the brain as a whole and the body as a whole are irreversibly dysfunctional, since the death of the brainstem entails both physical as well as psychological disintegration. In short, only a definition of death of the person which includes the death of the brainstem will meet Jonas's valid demand.

The concept of death which emphasises the death of the brainstem avoids the dualistic ambiguities inherent in formulations based on loss of hemispheric functions. Any valid criteria for death must consider the function of the body as a whole, not just the part of the brain with alleged responsibility for psychological responses. Death can only be determined in terms of a concept that specifies irreversible loss of bodily integration combined with the loss of any *capacity* for consciousness and cognition. Contemporary dualists, who see the cerebral hemispheres as synonymous with the soul or its psychological equivalent, are just as mistaken as their traditional predecessors. Against all forms of dualism it is necessary to reiterate Wittgenstein's objection to the conception of the human soul as a substance. 'The human body is the best picture of the human soul', wrote Wittgenstein in his *Philosophical Investigations* (II, iv) by which he meant that a human being is only human in the context of a capacity for physical functioning, however limited that might be. Brain cells growing in tissue culture have as little relation to human life as the various forms of disembodied consciousness that are cited by dualists. Philosophers' tales, and science fiction examples of Jones's and Smith's identity changes, ultimately require that if these beings are deemed to be alive their respective identities are located in bodies with human form and function. Furthermore there are no accounts of what Jones is, or where he is, or what he feels like, when he is transiting between bodies. Mental events require location in a human body, not in parts of a brain or soul.

At an elementary level it might be said that a person is dead when the possibility for having experience ceases. Taking the broadest definition of experience it would appear that this is when brainstem activity has permanently ceased. This is the point when the critical system has ceased to function and the body has entered the process of dissolution. Nevertheless, while death involves the permanent loss of experience, it does not follow that 'cessation of conscious experience' is an adequate criterion for a diagnosis of death. Life without conscious experience may be meaningless, possibly futile, but it does not amount to death.

These propositions would be disputed by philosophers who employ a concept of death based exclusively on the cessation of conscious experience. Thus Johnstone (1976, p. 220) argues that the relation between 'bodily dissolution' and 'death' is synthetic rather than analytic.

When the experiences of a person whose body has not yet dissolved have nonetheless permanently ceased it is not wholly metaphysical, I think, to speak of such a person undergoing a 'living death'. The fact that this phrase is not an outright contradiction shows, I think, that the relation between the dissolution of the body and the permanent cessation of experience is not one of strict equivalence.

The problem with Johnstone's argument is that to advance death to a point prior to that of loss of bodily integration is arbitrary and ambiguous. How, except through the loss of bodily integration, can we be certain that experience has permanently ceased? It may not be 'wholly metaphysical' to speak of a 'living death', but the boundaries of this concept are extremely hard to define and inevitably involve contentious theological and philosophical assumptions. Moreover, in some cases 'living deaths' can be reversed. This is why, if a clear and unambiguous criterion of death is required, it must involve concepts and criteria related to irreversible bodily disintegration.

The strictly biological concept of death, which has been advocated throughout this text, sees loss of personal identity, cognition and other properties associated with the hemispheric regions as concomitant of death, but not death itself. Diagnosing death is a biological, not a psychological, moral or a social task.

Conclusion

Death, so defined as the irreversible loss of function of the organism as a whole, is a singular concept. It does not make sense to speak of one kind of death for humans and another kind for other life forms. It may be the case that humans are the only species with a sense of personal identity, but the loss of this sense should not imply a different form of death for humans. A human being without identity is just as alive as any other living being.

Criteria for death based on an alleged loss of personal identity are unhelpful. They could imply support for proposals to diagnose death prior to loss of bodily integration. There are a number of states preceding death where it could be said that personal identity has been lost. A patient on a respirator, in a coma, may have lost his or her personal identity but still be alive. Loss of consciousness, loss of personal identity, do not necessarily involve strictly biological concepts, but death does. For ultimately the concept of 'death' can only be applied to organisms, not persons. Research in artificial intelligence may result in the creation of a person, (see Sloman, 1979) but the construction of an artificial corpse is an absurdity. As Culver and Gert (1982, p. 183) point out: 'The person in room 612 died last night' is only an indirect way of referring to the death of the organism that was that person. A person in a persistent vegetative state is just that: alive in the most basic biological sense.

9 ETHICS AND BRAIN DEATH

> There is nothing beyond his power. His subtlety meeteth all chance,
> all danger conquereth. For every ill he hath found its remedy, save
> only death.
>
> Sophocles, *Antigone*.

Introduction

The moral dilemmas related to sophisticated health-care technology
have not actually been caused by scientific advances in this area.
Instead, it might be said that the technology itself was a response to a
deeper and prior moral concern. Death is being increasingly seen in
terms of a disease to be conquered, and physicians have taken up the
challenge. To this extent the ethical problems of high technology can
be seen to arise, not merely as a by-product of that technology but as
consequences of a deeper moral problem regarding the meaning of
death. In the West, life has been given an intrinsic value, and a fatal-
istic acceptance of a predestined death has only a metaphorical
meaning. In this respect Dylan Thomas's poem entitled 'Do not go
gently into that good night' with its imperative to 'rage against the
dying of the light' epitomises contemporary medicine's obligation to
expand the boundaries of life. In response to this challenge medical
scientists seek wonder drugs, speak of immortality, and hint at eternal
youth. Developments in medical technology, and intensive care, stem
from a morally based desire to extend the span of human life. They
have generated further questions regarding the physician's ethical duties
and the patient's rights.

The possibility of extensive resuscitation has raised four distinct
questions which have been notoriously confused in medical literature:
(1) Is the patient dead? (2) Should the patient be allowed to die? (3)
When should resuscitation be discontinued? (4) When, and under what
circumstances, should decisions be taken with regard to the authorisation of the removal of organs? It is of the utmost importance to
recognise that these questions are fundamentally different in kind.

Is the Patient Dead?

Once the concept and criteria for human death have been clearly established this question becomes one of medical diagnosis. According to the concept of death so defined as the irreversible loss of integrated function of the organism as a whole, the patient is dead when tests have demonstrated that the brainstem has irreversibly ceased to function. Anything short of brainstem death, for example destruction of the hemispheric regions of the brain alone, is unacceptable. Damage confined to these regions does not satisfy the necessary and sufficient conditions for the death of a human being. Those who advocate the identification of the vegetative state (death of the cerebral hemispheres) with death are, whether they know it or not, asking for a change in the current homicide laws and could be seen to be 'asking for the introduction of euthanasia'. (see Horan, 1978, p. 365)

Should the Patient be Allowed to Die?

This question is bound up with the problem of prognosis and of the planning it implies. It calls for a comparison of alternatives. Whereas the scope of the first question is limited to objective clinical evidence, and draws upon established medical facts, this second question may involve ethical, religious and economic considerations, and may involve answers which reflect different moral attitudes towards the quality of residual life. Questions concerning whether the patient is alive or dead, like questions concerning pregnancy, or meningitis, demand a yes-no answer. But answers to the question 'Should the patient be allowed to die?' are not immediately clear-cut. They entail a consideration of a wide range of possibilities, ranging from the continuance of intensive life-support to the withdrawal of some, but not all, forms of treatment. When deciding if the patient is dead, deference to the expertise of the physician is needed. When deciding whether the patient should be allowed to die, one may have to refer to legal, ethical, economic and political matters, and one must take into consideration the known wishes of the patient, relatives and others. When the first question (is the patient dead?) has been answered affirmatively, the second question is obviously meaningless.

Distinctions between the two questions have not always been maintained. The Harvard Report of 1968 implicitly confused ventilation after brain death with the prolongation of life. The Report invoked the statement of Pope Pius XII to the effect that there was no obligation on the part of the physician to employ extraordinary measures to prolong life. But as the Task Force on Death and Dying of the Institute of Society, Ethics and the Life Sciences (1972) pointed out, this confused the factual question of the determination of death with the ethical question of when, if ever, a patient should be allowed to die.

A source of potential confusion between the two questions stems from the fact that 'switching off' the ventilator may appropriately follow an affirmative answer to either question. Nevertheless, the meaning of the action would differ in each situation. In the first situation the ventilator would be 'switched off' by the physician *after* an affirmative diagnosis of death. In the second situation 'switching off' would be an act of euthanasia and the onus of justification would rest with the physician concerned. In cases where brainstem function persists, 'switching off' is both unethical and possibly illegal.

The possibility of prolonged attempts at resuscitation raises the question of death with dignity. Must the patient be subjected to a hopeless and futile regime of intravenous alimentation or nasogastric tubes, dialysis, repeated sternal thumping, or electric shock to the chest, in order to survive for another day or week? Are a few statutory hours on the ventilator to become the last rite of modern medicine? Giving up when the prognosis is hopeless cannot be interpreted as a form of passive euthanasia. It cannot be a case of just 'allowing to die' since, if all treatment is 'hopeless', the physician is not in a position to allow the patient to die. All he can do is cease to apply a useless treatment. In such cases the choice facing the doctor is not whether to allow the patient to die, but *how* the patient shall die: either over a prolonged period in institutional isolation wired up to a mass of electronic gadgetry, or in relative dignity, possibly within a few hours or a day or two earlier. To discontinue treatment in hopeless cases is not 'letting die' but letting die in a more acceptable manner. The statement 'I let him die' only has meaning if it was ever possible at some stage to specify alternatives for maintaining life.

When Should Resuscitation be Discontinued?

Criteria for brain death are ethically necessary because it is possible to maintain organs alive in a cadaver when integrated life has ceased to be possible. Thus the moment when the brain has been determined to be dead is the moment when further resuscitation becomes pointless.

Korein (1978, p. 33) says that: 'To maintain the function of a brain-dead patient only because the technical means exist is a moral and economic atrocity that has evolved through a perversion of modern science.' Korein is obviously in favour of discontinuing ventilation or cardio-vascular support after brain death. But how a corpse is to be treated after death is a problem which affects relatives and social agencies as well as the physician. The physician has a primary duty to maintain life. Once he is satisfied beyond doubt that the patient is dead, he has no moral duty to ventilate a cadaver. If he is responsible for the mechanical respiratory system under his control, his duty is to disconnect and either save electricity or utilise the machine for another patient. To do so in this context is neither active nor passive euthanasia: 'Disconnecting the respirator should seem no more significant than drawing the sheet over a body once all the conditions for declaring brainstem death have been met.' (Pallis, 1980a)

Could problems arise if the relatives or responsible social agencies are willing to provide alternative means of ventilation, despite an assurance that the patient is dead? Should they be free to do so? Obviously this is not the kind of service that should be provided in a hospital, at the taxpayers' expense where those with responsibility for the care of patients have an ethical duty to ensure that facilities are kept available for the living and that hospital wards are not treated as mortuaries. Under these circumstances a decision by the relatives to continue ventilation would be a personal decision (with all the implications that entails) akin to a decision as to where to bury the body. A ventilated cadaver would not be alive, but 'treated as alive'. This might suggest immaturity among those responsible for the request, but possibly no more than embalming or mummification. It would, however, be considerably more expensive, and it is doubtful if the relatives in question could persuade physicians to undertake such a grisly task for long. When ventilation of the dead is carried out, as it still is in some cases, it is simply as a gesture to the relatives. Needless to say, none have ever recovered. (Jennett, 1980)

To what extent should a physician take into consideration concepts of death pertaining to another culture? In February 1983, the death of the Korean boxer Duk Koo Kim, was discussed in the *Hastings Center Report*. The young man had died of injuries sustained in the ring at Las Vegas in November 1983:

Nevada has a brain death statute, and the diagnosis was made shortly after the fight ended. Nevertheless, Duk Koo Kim was not immediately removed from the respirator. Instead efforts were made to determine the identity of his wife, and to have him treated by a Korean physician, who said, 'in the culture of the Korean people, Kim is still alive'. His attending physician is quoted as having said he would make a decision to disconnect the respirator consistent with 'the law, medical ethics, and the wishes of the family'. Later he called in a judge to 'protect' himself, and it was only when the patient was actually declared dead with the concurrence of the judge and the patient's family that the ventilator was finally removed. Public attention obviously was a more important determiner of action than Nevada's brain death statute. (Annas, 1983, p. 21)

Annas reported these facts to show that a brain-death statute has less importance for the attendant physician than public feelings and the wishes of the relatives. There is much to be said for this argument. The mere existence of a brain-death statute, however well defined, is not, of itself, a necessary or sufficient reason for the termination of resuscitative procedures. Certain cultural traditions may insist on the continuation of ventilation beyond the diagnosis of brain death. Provided that it is clearly indicated that the patient is dead, further ventilation should be seen in terms of procedures for dealing with corpses and equivalent to funeral rites, embalming and so on. If respect for the relatives' wishes, involves ventilation beyond brainstem death, this should not, under any circumstances be presented as a mode of life extension. Although ventilation to asystole (following brainstem death) may correspond with the wishes of the relatives, it is essential that the physician recognises and communicates the biological fact that death has occurred when tests have demonstrated that the brainstem is dead. A death certificate should be issued at this point to make things as explicit as possible. It is one thing to continue ventilation to asystole out of respect for a different cultural tradition, but an entirely different matter to reinforce ignorance and the beliefs that life is being maintained or extended.

Ventilation Following Maternal Brain Death

Some ethical confusion has been created by reports of maternal brain death occurring where brain death has occurred during pregnancy, with foetal survival depending on continued maternal circulation. In a report on foetal survival after maternal brain death, Dillon, Lee, Tronolone, Buckwald and Foote (1982) described a 26-week-old infant delivered by Caesarean section four days after its mother had been diagnosed as brain dead. The authors (p. 1091) outline the advantages of ventilation beyond death in terms of enhanced prospects of foetal survival: 'A foetus delivered at 25 weeks gestation has a 38% chance of survival that increases to 61% at 26 weeks and 76% at 27 weeks' gestation.' Given that maternal asystole may be delayed for two or three weeks after brain death, Dillon *et al.* suggested that vigorous management of the brain-dead mother prior to Caesarean section could substantially increase the prospects of foetal survival. The prognosis for pregnancies when the mother was in a vegetative state was even better.

The immediate consequence of proposals for maternal ventilation after brain death was the calling into question of what has been a matter of general agreement in medical literature 'that postmortem Caesarean section will not be successful and, therefore, is not justified if the pregnancy has not progressed beyond 28 weeks'. (Dillon *et al.*, 1982, p. 1090) The time that a foetus can be maintained in a brain-dead mother, despite vigorous management, is limited. On the most optimistic cardiac prognosis for the mother, one would be talking about days, rather than weeks. Of course this is not the case with the maintenance of a foetus whose mother is in a vegetative state. For example, Dillon *et al.* report on a case seen in 1977 involving a successful birth outcome in a case of prolonged post-traumatic coma, where 'the pregnancy was maintained from the sixth to the thirty-fourth week with the mother in a vegetative state'. (ibid. p. 1091) Brain dead mothers could not be maintained for such long periods. Nevertheless, Dillon *et al.* suggests that, if a patient is diagnosed brain dead (with a potentially viable foetus) between 24 and 27 weeks of gestation, then 'vigorous maternal support and foetal monitoring (should) be instituted'. (ibid.)

A clear-cut distinction between brain death and the vegetative state is extremely important when reaching decisions regarding the viability of the foetus. As Dillon *et al.* (ibid) conclude:

> Careful application of the definition of 'brain death' will allow the clinician an opportunity to preserve a favourable pregnancy outcome in the midst of some tragedies and to avoid futile, expensive attempts to preserve maternal life in others.

Maternal brain death highlights the significance of a clearly formulated definition of death *as an event* to be distinguished from the vegetative state, often referred to by philosophers and lay-persons as a 'lingering death'. Pregnancy in a vegetative state involves a situation where the mother is capable, with assistance, of sustaining the foetus to term; whereas foetal survival in a ventilated cadaver, following maternal brain death, is simply a situation where physicians are utilising the uterus of an ex-patient to enhance the probability of a favourable pregnancy outcome.

Nevertheless, foetal survival following maternal brain death has reinforced scepticism concerning the whole brain concept of death among some philosophers and physicians. In an editorial accompanying the report by Dillon *et al.* in the Sept. 3, 1982 issue of *Journal of the American Medical Association*, Siegler and Wikler suggest that foetal survival after brain death calls into question the claim that brain death provides a necessary and sufficient condition for diagnosing the death of the person as a whole.

> Now we are told that a brain-dead patient can nurture a child in the womb, which permits live birth several weeks 'postmortem'. Perhaps this is the straw which breaks the conceptual camel's back . . . The death of the brain seems not to serve as a boundary; it is a tragic, ultimately fatal loss, but not death itself. Bodily death occurs later, when integrated functioning ceases. (Siegler and Wikler, 1982, p. 1101)

The objection is wholly misleading. According to the brainstem concept of death, integrated functioning ceases with the irreversible cessation of brainstem function. If physicians continue to speak of 'brain-dead' patients being equivalent to 'terminally ill' patients, or as still possessing 'bodily life', or, as Dillon *et al.* do, of 'prolonging maternal life in the face of brain death', it means they have not yet fully grasped the concept of brainstem death. It does not indicate a problem with the definition of death itself, nor does it suggest shortcomings in the criteria by which brainstem death is diagnosed. Foetal survival following brainstem death of the mother is nothing more than foetal survival in a ventilated cadaver. It signifies no more 'life' in the ex-patient than embryonic survival in a test-tube would suggest that test-tubes or associated laboratory equipment were endowed with vital properties. In the case of maternal brain death reported by Dillon *et al.*, the artificial maintenance of certain organs (the womb) to support the foetus was nothing more than another form of mechanical support, equivalent to an incubator. The mother was not supporting the foetus anymore than one who, having bequeathed her organs, can be said to support the recipient after her death. The mother's organs were manipulated with the aid of sophisticated equipment, to maintain the life of the foetus. In this respect there is nothing different in this case from any other use of cadaver organs to sustain another life. Why should the uterus have greater significance than the heart or the kidneys of a cadaver? Given the possibility of more extensive means of salvaging corpses, one should remember that what is being managed in these cases is not patients but organs (the remnants of patients).

The issues raised in the discussion of maternal ventilation after brain death do not call into question the brainstem concept of death, nor do they introduce any new ethical problems concerning the management of patients. The ethical problems here belong to discussions concerning the disposal of organs after death or of the corpses themselves. According to USA legal procedures, if the patient had, under the provisions of The Uniform Anatomical Gift Act (UAGA), signed an anatomical donation card, then physicians could freely use her body as an incubator. If she had not, permission would have to be obtained from her next of kin. This raises the kind of ethical problem discussed by Veatch (1982, p. 1103) in response to Dillon's report. Suppose the next of kin does not want the organs of the pregnant brain-dead female maintained after her death. If she did not possess a UAGA card, then her organs cannot be used. But a complicating factor here might turn on the relationship of the woman to the father of the foetus. Legally, her marital spouse, as next of kin, would be decisively responsible for what happened to her organs and hence for the possible survival of the foetus. But an unmarried father of the foetus would have no such legal rights. And, as Veatch points out, to give him the authority to insist on the use of the woman's body against the wishes of her next of kin would require setting a precedent. Obviously this is an area where new ethical guidelines will have to be drawn. As Veatch points out, it is only by opening these discussions to many different disciplines that the richness of the issues will be fully appreciated. Hearing the views of clinicians is important, but clinical expertise cannot establish how a society should classify an ex-patient, or how he or she should be treated in terms of ethics or the law.

Neomorts and Organ Banks

The possibility of maintaining the circulation for a while after brain death has given rise to ethical concern regarding the employment of cadavers as organ banks. Gaylin, (1974) for example, expresses a strong ethical resistance to the view that the newly-dead could be used as a kind of resource. He points out that, whilst a diagnosis of brain death may enable a physician to terminate treatment without the accusation of euthanasia, it nevertheless creates other problems. If one grants the right to 'pull the plug', one also grants the privilege not to do so. Gaylin raises the spectre of cadavers having the legal status of being dead but having some of the qualities associated with life: they would be warm, pulsating and urinating. To be useful they would require nursing, and provided that was of a high quality they could be maintained in that state for some time. Gaylin describes these cadavers as 'neomorts' − newly deceased bodies which are maintained in a state of cellular viability for the purpose of organ transplantation. Gaylin (1974, p. 30) sees this as a form of moral corruption, for he writes: 'Sustaining life is an urgent argument for any measure, but not if that measure destroys those very qualities that make life worth sustaining.'

Gaylin is concerned that the employment of brain-related criteria for diagnosing death may lead down the slippery slope to other surgical assaults on the newly dead. His argument can be presented as follows. (1) With brain-related criteria for death one is obliged to maintain the patient on a respirator until a diagnosis of death has been made. (2) It is acceptable to keep the respirator going until the organs are removed for transplantation purposes. These two steps are relatively innocuous. But why, he asks, is it necessary to turn the respirator off, in a brain dead patient if there are no immediate demands for transplant organs? At this point moral objections are expressed. Walton (1980, p. 37) summarises them:

> The ventilated cadaver could be used as a bank for other organs or a plant for manufacturing biochemical compounds. It could be used as a self-replenishing blood-bank or for surgical and grafting research. Even further, it could be used for immunological research or testing new drugs. Finally, even medical instruction is included as a possibility.

Like Gaylin, Walton presents the above account as the hypothetical endstage of an ethical slippery slope. He maintains that these possibilities need not become actualities: there is no necessary rule which says that every possibility must become an actuality. The proponent of the slippery slope argument must provide additional evidence to show how the feasible could become fact. This is relatively easy. The use of ventilated cadavers does not involve any radical departure from existing practices. Frozen organs have been employed ever since techniques of freezing and preservation of organs were developed. People who freely donate their bodies for research do so in that knowledge. It is a short and logical step from there to the employment of more refined techniques of preservation, including ventilators. Admittedly, the idea of vaults of 'neomorts', as presented by Gaylin, is a rather grisly extension of this. And if it were feasible it might lead down a slope on which it would be hard to maintain one's grip. But any steps in that direction are not the result of an acceptance of brain-related criteria for death. The possibilities only arise because of the availability of respirator technology, which can maintain cadaver organs for a limited period more efficiently than techniques of freezing. Criteria for death are one matter; the slope begins at the point where attitudes towards the newly-dead begin to change. Techniques for mummification and embalming have been available for centuries. In a climate of changing attitudes towards the newly-dead, there might be the possibility of a gradual shift of attitudes from the acceptance of ventilated cadavers as organ banks to acceptance of public displays of animated cadavers, resembling a macabre exhibition of animated dolls. But this would not be due to the evolution of technology. It would be due to a sinister evolution of cultural attitudes. Ventilators and other associated techniques of organ preservation are a response to a moral need. They do not generate this need. There may develop a measure of public acceptability for the display of animated corpses just as it is today acceptable to display a resting Lenin in Red Square, or Jeremy Bentham in Bedford College. The fact that a machine can ventilate corpses does open up macabre possibilities, but these are not generated in any way by neurological criteria for diagnosing death.

There are, however, very strong ethical imperatives concerning the newly-dead. To be declared dead is to be beyond the scope of ethical imperatives regarding treatment. But after a diagnosis of death, the ex-patient still has a number of rights and moral obligations, including the right to proper interment, to the distribution of his or her property according to known wishes and to a whole network of manifestations of respect for the corpse. Even laboratory cadavers in a mortuary or post mortem room are not supposed to be treated as lumps of flesh, and ethical imperatives governing their disposal are as strict as any which apply to the living. Ethical attitudes of respect for the body of the deceased may change, but this change will be independent of any shift in the criteria for determining whether the person is dead. A corpse is entitled to certain rights which are independent of whether parts of the body are maintained in a state of cellular life on a ventilator, or of whether the deceased is a skeleton or just the ashes left by an explosion which has destroyed its human form. In none of the latter cases can we be said to be given a living person rights; we are simply acknowledging what is due to an ex-person. The fact that a brain-dead ex-patient resembles a living person is not a reason for blurring the distinction between life and death. The resemblance to a living person should not imply (or demand) the same status as that person. We can see this if we consider whether it would be worse to mutilate the corpse or a lifelike wax replica of the person. Apart from those instances where the destruction of a statue or picture is a way of attacking the power of a dead person, it would generally be considered more unacceptable to mutilate the corpse. This applies even in cases where the remains bear no resemblance to the ex-person, as in an air crash, explosion or fire.

When, and Under What Circumstances, Should Decisions be Taken With Regard to the Authorisation of the Removal of Organs?

Tremendous pressure exists for more transplant donors, and these pressures will grow. A physician can be subjected to conflicting moral obligations when the organs in one patient can be used to save the life of another. To avoid potential conflicts between the attending physician and the requirements of the transplant team, practices have been evolved which ensure that the donor's physician should have no role in the transplantation procedure itself. For this reason the Judicial Council of the American Medical Association requires that the donor's death be determined by someone other than the recipient's physician. Similarly, the Committee on Morals and Ethics of the Transplantation Society of the USA says that 'acceptance of death should be made and declared by at least two physicians whose primary responsibility is care of the potential donor and is independent of the transplant team'. (Black, 1978, p. 397)

Since artificially maintained bodies present a new entity for the law and society, the President's Commission was mandated to 'study and recommend ways in which the traditional legal standards can be updated in order to provide clear and principled guidance for determining whether such bodies are alive or dead'. (*DD*, 1981, p. 3) Essential to the mandate was the premiss that any statutory definition of death should be kept separate and distinct from provisions governing the donation of cadaver organs, and from any legal rules about decisions to terminate life-sustaining treatment. Despite criticism of the facts, the majority of patients diagnosed as brain dead do not become organ donors. The President's Commission referred to 36 comatose patients who were declared dead on the basis of irreversible loss of brain function, but of these only six became organ donors. According to the report: (*DD*, 1981, p. 24)

> medical concern over the determination of death . . . rests much less with any wish to facilitate organ transplantation than with the need both to render appropriate care to patients and to replace artificial support with more fitting and respectful behaviour when a patient has become a dead body.

Having clearly outlined the legal and moral status of criteria for brain death, one can then, and only then, justify decisions regarding the re-use of cadaver organs. According to Veith *et al.*, (1977, p. 1745) a clearly defined statute on brain death would permit the physician 'to cooperate in efforts to procure cadaver organs in optimal conditions for transplantation into other patients'. It is, however, important that proposals for statutes on brain death should avoid the very serious risk of running together criteria for brain death with legislation for the removal of organs. For example, in 1976 the European Committee on Legal Cooperation fell into exactly this trap when it supported the following two positions:

(1) It should be possible for the removal of cadaver organs to be effected from the moment when it was established that the donor had irreversibly lost all his cerebral functions even though the function of other organs might have been preserved.
(2) Legislation should move towards the adoption of presumed consent for the removal of cadaver organs if circumstances give reason to believe that the family of the donor do not or would not have objected. (Cited by Walton, 1980, p. 13)

These two statements illicitly bring together proposals for brain-related criteria of death and legislation permitting the removal of cadaveric organs. The proposals are then linked with the particularly dangerous attempt to shift the burden for permission regarding the removal of cadaveric organs.

Confusion of this sort stems from earlier attempts to assimilate the phenomenon of brain death. The reasons why a definition of brain death was necessary were presented in terms of factors extraneous to the patient's welfare. The Harvard Report (1968), for example, gave two practical reasons for a redefinition of death:

(1)   Relief of the patient, kin, and medical resources from the burden of indefinitely prolonged coma.
(2)   Removal of controversy with regard to the obtaining of organs for transplantation.

In so far as the primary rationale behind the redefinition of death was to enable a physician to terminate treatment when it was no longer of any value to the patient there is nothing objectionable. There is, clearly, a strong ethical imperative to reduce the period of anxiety for relatives. There have been cases of relatives paying over $2000 a day to keep a corpse ventilated. (*DD*, 1981, p. 24)

However, objections to the second reason given in the Harvard Report have been raised by Hans Jonas who argues (1974, p. 133) that freedom for organ use is not covered by the primary rationale, that is, the interests of the patient. Jonas's point is that the theoretical requirement to define death is one thing, and it is essential if the patient's interests are uppermost. But the requirement for organ transplants — even to save lives — is another interest, one which must not be allowed to intrude upon the former. Commenting on the Harvard interest in organ transplants, Jonas (p. 133) says:

I contend that, pure as this interest, viz, to save other lives, is in itself, its intrusion into the *theoretical* attempt to define death makes the attempt impure; the Harvard Committee should never have allowed itself to adulterate the purity of its scientific case by baiting it with the prospect of this *extraneous* — though extremely appealing gain.

Jonas's concern is not with theoretical purity for its own sake. He is worried about the policy consequences of this impurity, once a need for the harvesting of organs is built into the definition of death. Stories about 'human vegetables' lingering on for months, when their organs could be used to save other lives, must never be allowed to influence criteria for determining death. Wherever such arguments occur they must be seen as advocacy for euthanasia or dissection of the living and their pros and cons evaluated. The fact that other humans might be capable of benefiting from organs extracted from patients in persistent vegetative states is no reason for assimilating these states with death. Discussions regarding the worth of a life should not replace discussions about the *existence* of a life. The term 'vegetative state' refers to the condition of a living being; there is no way in which it can be seen as anything other than an instance of life. It is clearly important to define death precisely in order to indicate when it may be possible to seek authorisation to harvest cadaver organs. But this is intrinsically different from a situation where the need for cadaver organs is allowed to interfere with judgements concerning the moment of death.

BRAIN DEATH AND THE SLIPPERY SLOPE

If the physician presumes to take into consideration in his work whether a life has value or not, the consequences are boundless and the physician becomes the most dangerous man in the state.

Dr Christoph Hufeland (1762-1836).

Brain Death and States Approaching Death

Throughout the preceding chapters it has been argued that the concept of brain death, with its heavy emphasis on the brainstem, is theoretically and practically superior to any other concept of death. It has been argued that 'higher brain' formulations provide necessary but not sufficient grounds for the diagnosis of death. From the ethical standpoint a failure to retain the distinction between a concept which specifies irreversible loss of brainstem function and 'higher brain' formulations can be seen to lead down a slippery slope where factual uncertainty regarding the moment of death may let in decisions to terminate treatment according to cost-benefit criteria and/or other utilitarian or extraneous considerations.

It has also been argued that human death is nothing less than the death of the organism as a whole, which can be established by tests for a permanently non-functioning brainstem. States approaching this condition may indicate imminent death, but not death itself. Nevertheless it is very easy to confuse the prediction of death with a diagnosis of death, as the following extract (Walton, 1980, p. 51) reveals:

Because the case for whole brain death admits of well-established, and widely corroborated criteria, with a clear clinical picture of pathological destruction that irreversibly and inevitably leads to death in a short time, we can see how it is much less open to the slippery slope refutations than the case for cerebral death.

Walton is correct in pointing out that the 'whole brain' formulation avoids the slippery slope charge. But he has inadvertently reintroduced the slope by depicting 'whole brain' death as a state which 'inevitably leads to death'. This must mean that whole brain death is not death, but a state prior to death. Drinking a litre of suphuric acid will lead inevitably to death. So will leaping out of an aeroplane without a parachute. These are not states of death; they are preludes to death. The point of whole brain formulations is that they are intended to determine the *state*, not the imminence of death. For this reason the slippery-slope argument is highly relevant when applied to the slipshod equating of 'going to die' with 'not going to recover', and 'virtually dead' with 'is dead'. Patients suffering permanent damage to the cerebral hemispheres may not recover, and from some ethical standpoints may be 'virtually dead', but they may not actually be dying, and provided they still possess a viable brainstem they are certainly not dead. An example of the apallic syndrome (another name for the persistent vegetative state) will illustrate this point.

In 1960, a young woman suffered an epileptic attack during pregnancy, followed by deep coma and transient cardio-respiratory failure. The EEG remained isolectric for the next 17 years. But her breathing remained spontaneous, and her pulse was regular. She retained movements of hands and feet, chewing and swallowing, withdrawal reflexes, and the capacity to respond to certain signals. She eventually died of a heart disease. 'The autopsy showed a shrunken brain with atrophied cerebral hemispheres transformed into thin-walled yellow-brown bags. The cerebral cortex was almost totally destroyed.' (Walton, 1980, p. 78) She was 'as good as dead', but she was very much alive because her critical system, the brainstem remained functional and capable of maintaining bodily integration.

The more severe forms of the vegetative state have been equated by some, with the death of the person. (Puccetti, 1976) In such a state the patient may be permanently unresponsive but able to breathe spontaneously and exhibit reflex actions, thus passing the Harvard tests for being alive. Many physicians, if not all, would find the idea of burial in this state inconceivable. Puccetti (1976, p. 252) does not:

All I can say to this is that it is not inconceivable to me. When reasonably assured of the loved one's neocortical death, it would not have the slightest interest for me that this person was still breathing when prepared for burial, however grisly it might seem to those who have to do that. And I should hope those close to me would feel the same in my own case. If someone suggested that my body might survive death of the neocortex for several months or years, provided it was fed and cleaned properly, etc. that would have no greater appeal to me than preservation of my appendix in a bottle of formaldehyde. For in the sense in which life has a value for human beings, I would have been dead all that time. And if the notion of burying a breathing corpse is repulsive, then I suggest we stop it from breathing.

This should be read as a proposal for euthanasia, not as an argument about the diagnosis of death. The objections to Puccetti's thesis are twofold. First, if we can bury a breathing patient just because his cerebral cortex has ceased to function then what safeguards are there against even earlier burial? Second, and perhaps more significantly, Puccetti's argument rests on a confusion between 'meaningful life functions' and 'the presence of life'. The former involves philosophical and moral components relating to the meaning and worth of life; the latter is primarily medical and related to the criteria for irreversible cessation of bodily integration. Even if one accepts that irreversible loss of the content of consciousness (the vegetative state) constitutes the death of the person as a whole — and it has been argued throughout this book that there are major objections to this — there would still be insurmountable problems in the attempt to determine whether all cognitive sentient activity ceased with the destruction of the cortex. A number of German researchers have argued that brainstem activity may be responsible for some primitive forms of psychic activity. (Horan, 1978, p. 367)

In an atmosphere of staggering health expenditure and cost-conscious welfare agencies there is a very real danger that pressure will be put on physicians to divert their energies from care of vegetative and noncognitive patients to other more immediate cases. Any discussion of this sort must be seen as an economic, ethical, political and legal matter which is distinct from the factual matter of determining the moment of death. It is important, therefore, to resist arguments which do not recognise the differences between the vegetative state and brain death. For there are philosophers, relying exclusively on psychological criteria for human personhood, who blur this distinction and unwittingly lend support to irresponsible Government agencies eager to avoid moral censure for termination of the treatment of certain categories of patients. Discussions in the press and elsewhere have expressed concern over the cost of caring for brain-damaged patients. However, there is a vast difference between the cost of management of brain-dead ex-patients and those in a vegetative state. One should be very cautious when reading muddled reports of staggering bills for the ventilation of cadavers which are sometimes presented as grounds for euthanasia in the persistent vegetative stage. Whilst the management of brain-dead ex-patients may require short-term maintenance, including total respirator support to retain cardiac function and circulation while any organs are harvested, patients in persistent vegetative states need considerable, long-term nursing care, although after the initial period they require much less medical attention.

Conclusion

The brainstem concept of death, which has been advocated throughout this text, maintains that bodily integration, which is dependent upon a viable brainstem, is constitutive of human life. Death of the brainstem can be determined by empirical tests.

Whilst the vegetative state is often cited as an example of a condition in which the patient may be allowed to die, philosophers who confuse or equate this state with brain death are taking the first step along a problem of factually diagnosing death on to a very dangerous slippery slope that leads to euthanasia. Uncertainty regarding criteria for determining the loss of hemispheric functions — for instance, the limited reliability of the EEG as a positive indicator — suggest that redefinitions of death in this direction run into serious risks of confusing criteria for euthanasia with criteria for diagnosing death. The first is an ethical issue with serious legal implications, the latter a clinical issue to be resolved by clinical expertise.

In a context of escalating health-care costs it is inevitable that there will be proposals to limit heroic and expensive methods of prolonging life. Persistent failure to present a clear-cut boundary between life and death may lend support to proposals for the termination of treatment according to cost-benefit criteria or on other extraneous grounds. But, if the doctor is not to be seen as an executioner, criteria for the termination of treatment must be based on a clearly defined, widely publicised, philosophically acceptable, and practically meaningful concept of death, not on a prognosis that death is imminent or on an estimate that residual life would be worthless. For this reason the definition of death, outlined and defended throughout this text, must be completely distinct from all other considerations.

BIBLIOGRAPHY

Agich, George J. (1976) 'The Concept of Death and Embodiment', *Ethics in Science and Medicine. 1*, 95-105

Agrist, A. (1958) 'Certified Cause of Death – Analysis and Recommendations', *Journal of the American Medical Association (JAMA)*, 26 Apr. *166*, 17, 2148-53

Annas. George J. (1983) 'Death: There Ought to be a Law', *Hastings Center Report. 13*, 1 (Feb.), 20-1

Anon. (1968) 'Criteria for Heart Transplants', *British Medical Journal (BMJ)* 23 Mar. *1*, 762

—— (1980) *BMJ*, 13 Oct. *231*, 1028

Aries, Phillipe (1976) *Western Attitudes Towards Death From the Middle Ages to the Present*, Marion Boyors, London

Arnold, John D. , Zimmerman, Thomas F. and Martin, Daniel, C. (1968) 'Public Attitudes and the Diagnosis of Death', *JAMA*, Nov., *206*, 9, 1949-54

Becker, D.P., Robert, C.M. and Nelson, J.R. (1970) 'An Evaluation of the Definition of Cerebral Death', *Neurology* (Minneapolis), *20*, 459-62

Becker, L.C. (1982) 'Human Being: The Boundaries of the Concept' in M. Cohen, T. Nagel and T. Scanlon (eds.), *Medicine and Moral Philosophy, A Philosophy and Public Affairs Reader*, Princeton University Press, New York, pp. 23-48

Beresford, H.R. (1978) 'Cognitive Death: Differential Problems and Legal Overtones', *Annals of New York Academy of Sciences, 315*, 339-48

Bernat, James L., Culver, Charles, M. and Gert, Bernard (1981) 'On the Definition and Criterion of Death', *Annals of Internal Medicine, 94*, 3, 389-94

Bertalanffy, L. von (1967) *General Systems Theory*, Penguin, Harmondsworth

Black, Peter McL. (1978) 'Brain Death', *New England Journal of Medicine*, 17 Aug., *299*, 338-44, 24 Aug. *299*, 393-401

Bolton, C.F. (1976) 'EEG and Brain Life', *Lancet*, 6 Mar., p. 535.

Boshes, B. (1978) 'Death: Historical Evolution and Implication of the Concept' in J. Korein (ed.), *Annals of the New York Academy of Sciences*, New York, *315*, 11-18

Browne, A. (1983) 'Whole Brain Death Reconsidered', *Journal of Medical Ethics, 9*, 28-31

Braunstein, P., Korein, J., Kricheff, I. and Lieberman, A. (1978) 'Evaluation of the Critical Deficit of Cerebral Circulation Using Radioactive Tracers (Bolus Technique'), *Annals of the New York Academy of Sciences, 315*, 143-67

Byrne, P., O'Reilly, S. and Quay, P.M. (1979) 'Brain Death: An Opposing Viewpoint', *JAMA*, 2 Nov., *242*, 18, 1985-90

Capron, A.M. and Kass, L.R. (1980) 'A Statutory Definition of the Standards for Determining Human Death', *University Pennsylvania Law Review, 121* (1972), 87-118; also in D.J. Horan and D. Mall (eds.), *Death, Dying and Euthanasia*, Aletheia, Maryland, 1980, pp. 40-74 (all references to the latter edition)

Churchill, Larry R. (1979) 'Interpretation of Dying: Ethical Implications for Patient Care', *Ethics in Science and Medicine*, o, 211-22

Collins, Vincent J. (1980) 'Considerations in Prolonging Life: A Dying and Recovery Score' in D.J. Horan and D. Mall (eds.), *Death, Dying and Euthanasia*, Aletheia, Maryland, pp. 3-26

Committee on Irreversible Coma and Brain Death (1978) *Transactions of the American Neurological Association, 103*, 320-1

Conference of Medical Royal Colleges and Their Faculties in the United Kingdom (1976) 'Diagnosis of Brain Death', *BMJ* Nov., *2*, 1187-8

—— (1979) 'Diagnosis of Death', *BMJ*, Feb., *1*, 3320

Cranford, Ronald E. and Smith, Harman L. (1979) 'Some Critical Distinctions between Brain Death and the Persistent Vegetative State', *Ethics in Science and Medicine, 6*, 199-209

Culver, C.M. and Gert, B. (1982) *Philosophy in Medicine: Conceptual and Ethical Issues in Medicine and Psychiatry*, Oxford University Press, Oxford

De Mere, M. and Alexander, T. (1975) 'Report on Definitions of Death from the Law and Medicine Committee', *Chicago American Bar Association*, 25 Feb. 1975

Dillon, William P., Lee, Richard V., Tronolone, Michael J., Buckwald, Sharon and Foote, Ronald J. (1982) 'Life Support and Maternal Brain Death during Pregnancy', *JAMA* 3 Sept., *248*, 9, 1089-91

Earl, A. (1974) 'The Death of a Brain', *Johns Hopkins Medical Journal, 124*, 190-201

Engelhardt Jr., H. Tristam (1971) 'Splitting the Brain, Dividing the Soul, Being of Two Minds: An Editorial concerning Mind-Body Quandaries in Medicine', *Journal of Medicine and Philosophy, 2*, 2, 89-100

Executive Committee of the Netherlands Red Cross Society (1970) Third International Congress of the Transplantation Society, *A Memorandum on Organ Transplantation*, The Hague

Fox, R.F. and Swazey, J.P. (1974) *The Courage to Fail*, University Chicago Press, Chicago

Friloux Jr, C. Anthony (1980) 'Death, When Does It Occur?' in D.J. Horan and D. Mall (eds.), *Death, Dying and Euthanasia*, Aletheia, Maryland, pp. 27-38

Gaylin, W. (1974) 'Harvesting the Dead', *Harpers*, 23 Sept., *249*, 23-46

Gert, Bernard (1971) 'Personal Identity and the Body', *Dialogue, 10*, 458-78

Green, M.B. and Wikler, D. (1982) 'Brain Death and Personal Identity' in M. Cohen, T. Nagel and T. Scanlon, (eds.), *Medicine and Moral Philosophy*, Princeton University Press, New Jersey, pp. 49-77

Harth, Eric (1982) *Windows on the Mind*, Harvester, Brighton

Harvard Medical School (1968) 'A Definition of Irreversible Coma', *JAMA*, 5 Aug., *205*, 6, 85-8

Hauerwas, Stanley (1979) 'Reflections on Suffering, Death and Medicine', *Ethics in Science and Medicine, 6*, 229-37

Hegel, G.W.F. (1904) *The Logic of Hegel*, trans. by W. Wallace, Oxford University Press, Oxford

High, Dallas M. (1972) 'Death: Its Conceptual Elusiveness', *Soundings*, Winter

Hodges, Louis W. (1979) 'Third-Party Payment and Treatment of the Dying Patient', *Ethics in Science and Medicine, 6*, 223-8

Horan, D.J. (1978) 'Euthanasia and Brain Death: Ethical and Legal Considerations', *Annals New York Academy of Sciences, 315*, 363-75

Ibe, K. (1971) 'Clinical and Pathophysiological Aspects of the Intravital Brain

Death', *Electroencephalogr. Clinical Neurophysiology, 30*, 272

Ingvar, D.H., Arne, B., Johansson, L. and Samuelsson, S.M. (1978) 'Survival after Severe Cerebral Anoxia with Destruction of the Cerebral Cortex: The Apallic Syndrome', *Annals New York Academy of Sciences, 315*, 184-214

Jennett, B. (1980) quoted in an editorial, *BMJ*, 6 Dec. *281*, 1509

—— and Plum, F. (1972) 'The Persistent Vegetative State: A Syndrome in Search of a Name', 1 Apr., *Lancet*, 734-7

Johnstone Jr, Henry W. (1976) 'Sleep and Death', *Monist*, Apr. *59*, 2, 218-33

—— (1978) 'Does Death have a Nature?', *Journal of Medicine and Philosophy, 3*, 1, 8-23

Jonas, Hans (1974) 'Against the Stream: Comments on the Definition and Redefinition of Death', *Philosophical Essays: From Ancient Creed to Technological Man*, Prentice Hall, Engelwood Cliffs, NJ

Jørgensen, E.O. (1973) 'Spinal Man after Brain Death', *Acta Neurochirurogica, 28*, 259-73

Kass, L.R. (1977) 'Death Process or Event? A Reply to Morison', *Science, 173* (1971), 698-702; also in R.F. Weir (ed.), *Ethical Issues in Death and Dying*, Columbia University Press, New York, 1977, pp. 69-74 (all quotes are taken from the latter publication)

Kaste, Markku, Hillbom, Matti and Palo, Jorma (1979) 'Diagnosis and Management of Brain Death', *BMJ*, 24 Feb. 1, 525-7

Kennedy, Ian (1971) 'The Kansas Statute on Death: An Appraisal', *New England Journal of Medicine, 285*, 946-50

Korein, J. (1978) 'The Problem of Brain Death', *Annals of the New York Academy of Sciences, 315*, 19-38

—— and Maccario, M. (1971) 'On the Diagnosis of Cerebral Death: A Prospective Study of 55 Patients to Define Irreversible Coma', *Clinical Electroencephalograph, 2*, 178-99

Ladd, John (1979) 'The Definition of Death and the Right to Die' in J. Ladd (ed.), *Issues Relating to Life and Death*, Oxford University Press, Oxford, pp. 118-45

Lamb, D. (1978) 'Diagnosing Death', *Philosophy and Public Affairs*, Winter, 7, 2, 144-53

—— (1979) *Hegel: From Foundation to System*, Nijhoff, The Hague

Lunde, D.T. (1969) 'Psychiatric Complications of Heart Transplants', *American Journal of Psychiatry*, Sept. *126*, 3, 369-73

Lynn, Joanne (1983) 'The Determination of Death', *Annals of Internal Medicine*, Aug., *99*, 2, 264-6

MacGillivray, B. (1980) quoted by T. Smith in 'Medicine and the Media', *BMJ*, 29 Nov. *281*, 1485

McWhirter, N. (ed.), (1981) *The Guinness Book of Records*, Bantam, New York

Medawar, J.S. and Medawar, P.B. (1978) *The Life Sciences*, Paladin, London

Morison, R.S. (1977) 'Death: Process or Event?', *Science, 173* (1971), 694-8, also in R.F. Weir (ed.), *Ethical Issues in Death and Dying*, Columbia University Press, New York, 1977, pp. 57-69 (all quotes are from the latter publication)

Mollaret, P., and Goulon, M. (1959) 'Le Coma Dépassé', *Revue Neurologie, 101*, 3-15

Natanson, Maurice (1978) 'The Nature of Death: Editorial and Bibliography',

116 *Bibliography*

Journal of Medicine and Philosophy, Mar. *3*, 1, 1-7

National Institute of Neurological and Communicative Disorders (NINCDS Collaborative Study 1977) 'An Appraisal of the Criteria of Cerebral Death', *JAMA*, 17 Mar. *237*, 10, 982-6

Ouaknine, G.I.Z., Kosary, J., Braham, P. Czerniak and Hillel, N. (1973) 'Laboratory Criteria of Brain Death', *Journal of Neurosurgery, 39*, 429-33

Pallis, C. (1980a) quoted in 'News and Notes', *BMJ*, 1 Nov. *281*, 1220

—— (1980b) Letter, *Lancet*, 15 Nov., p. 1085

—— (1983a) *The ABC of Brainstem Death*, British Medical Journal, London

—— (1983b) 'Whole Brain Death Reconsidered – Physiological Facts and Philosophy', *Journal of Medical Ethics, 9*, 32-7

—— and MacGillivray, B. (1980) 'Brain Death and the EEG', *Lancet*, 15 Nov., 1085-6

—— and Prior, P.F. (1983) 'Guidelines for the Determination of Death', *Neurology*, Feb., *33*, 251

Parfit, D. (1971) 'Personal Identity', *The Philosophical Review, 80*, 3-27

Poole, E. (1980) Letter, *BMJ*, 1 Nov., *281*, 1213

Pope Pius XII (1958) 'The Prolongation of Life', An Address of Pope Pius XII to an International Congress of Anesthesiologists, 24 Nov. 1957; *The Pope Speaks*, 4 Nov. 1958

Posner, J.B. (1978) 'Coma and Other States of Consciousness: The Differential Diagnosis of Brain Death', *Annals New York Academy of Sciences, 315*, 339-48

Powner, David J. (1976) 'Drug-Associated Isoelectric EEG's: A Hazard in Brain Death Certification', *JAMA*, Sept., *236*, 10, 1123

President's Commission for the Study of Ethical Problems in Medicine and Biomedical and Behavioral Research (1981) *Defining Death*, Washington

Prior, Pamela F. (1980) 'Brain Death', *Lancet*, Nov., 1142

Puccetti, R. (1976) 'The Conquest of Death', *Monist, 59*, 2, 249-63

Rachels, James (1980) 'Euthanasia', *Matters of Life and Death*, Temple University Press, Philadelphia

Roelofs, R. (1978) 'Some Preliminary Remarks on Brain Death', *Annals New York Academy of Sciences, 315*, 39-44

Rot, Anne and van Till, H.A.H. (1971) 'Neocortical Death after Cortical Arrest', *Lancet*, Nov., 1099-100

Safar, Peter (1977) 'Resuscitation of the Arrested Brain in P.J. Safar and J.O. Elam (eds.), *Advances in Cardiopulmonary Resuscitation*, Springer Verlag, New York, pp. 177-81

Schiffer, R.B. (1978) 'The Concept of Death: Tradition and Alternative', *Journal of Medicine and Philosophy, 3*, 1, 24

Siegler, Mark and Wikler, Daniel (1982) 'Brain Death and Live Birth', editorial, *JAMA*, 3 Sept. *248*, 9, 1101-2

Sloman A. (1979) *The Computer Revolution in Philosophy*, Harvester, Brighton

Smith, Tony (1980) 'Medicine and the Media', *BMJ*, 29 Nov., *281*, 1485

Stickel, D.L. (1979) 'The Brain Death Criterion of Human Death', *Ethics in Science and Medicine, 6*, 4, 177-97

Task Force on Death and Dying of the Institute of Society, Ethics and the Life Sciences (1977) 'Refinements in Criteria for the Determination of Death: An Appraisal' in R.F. Weir (ed.), *Ethical Issues in Death and Dying*, Columbia

University Press, New York, pp. 90-102

Trammell, Richard L. (1978) 'The Presumption Against Taking Life', *Journal of Medicine and Philosophy*, *3*, 1, 53-67

Twycross, Robert (1979) 'Decisions About Dying and Death' in G. Scorer and A. Wing (eds.), *Decision Making in Medicine*, Edward Arnold, London, pp. 101-15

Veatch, R.M. (1978a) *Death, Dying and the Biological Revolution*, Yale University Press, New Haven

—— (1978b) 'The Definition of Death: Ethical, Philosophical, and Policy Confusion', *Annals New York Academy of Sciences, 315*, 307-21

—— (1982) 'Maternal Brain Death: An Ethicist's Thoughts', *JAMA*, 3 Sept., *248*, 9, 1102-3

Veith, Frank J., Fein, Jack M., Tendler, Moses D., Veatch, Robert M., Kleimon, Marc A., and Kalkines, George (1977) 'Brain Death: A Status Report', *JAMA*, 17 Oct. *238*, 16, 1744-8

Vesey, G. and Parfit D. (1974) 'Discussion' in G. Vesey (ed.), *Philosophy in the Open*, Open University Press, Milton Keynes, pp. 54-66

Wainwright-Evans, D. and Lum, L.C. (1980) Letter, *Lancet*, 8 Nov. 1022

Walton, D.N. (1980) *Brain Death*, Purdue University Press, Indiana

Whitwham, J.G. (1980) Letter, *Lancet*, 22 Nov., 1142

Youngner, S.J. and Bartlett, E.T. (1983) 'Human Death and High Technology: The Failure of the Whole Brain Formulations', *Annals of Internal Medicine*, *99*, 252-8

NAME INDEX

SUBJECT INDEX

anencephalic 14-15, 67, 85
angiography 51, 53-4, 64-7
apallic syndrome 110,115; *see
   also* vegetative state
apnoea 4, 5, 29 65
asystole 35-6, 48, 54-9, 99-100
autolysis 60

Collaborative Study 63, 67
Coma dépassé 4, 52
Conference of Medical Royal
   Colleges 5, 41, 48-9, 57, 66, 68,
   69, 114
consciousness 3, 5, 7, 11-12, 14,
   42-5, 48-9, 87, 91-3
critical system 7, 14, 16-17, 33-40,
   50, 80, 92, 110

decapitation 30, 46, 84
drug intoxication 48, 59-60, 63-8
dualism 58, 90-3

EEG 10, 51, 53-4, 64-9, 110, 112
entelechy 80
euthanasia 6, 8, 44, 56, 60, 95-7,
   103, 107-8, 111

Harvard Report 4, 15, 53-4, 62, 65,
   69, 96-7, 106-7
hypothermia 59, 63

irreplaceable 7, 34-5, 37-8
irreversible 2, 5, 7, 13-15, 19, 24-7,
   30, 33-4, 48, 58-63, 82-3, 93,
   106, 109

Kansas statute 20-3, 28

Law Reform Commission of Canada
   31

neomorts 102-5

Panorama Report 65-6, 68
personal identity 6, 7, 39, 42-4, 62,
   83-94, 111
pregnancy 99-102, 110

President's Commission 24-8, 31-2,
   39, 41, 46-7, 49-50, 60, 85-6,
   105-7
putrefaction 14, 36, 51, 74, 77, 79

reductionism 9, 38, 58, 66, 90
religion 2-4, 8, 11, 13-14, 58
resurrection 12, 88
resuscitation 2, 6, 18, 26, 30, 48, 59,
   64, 74, 77, 79, 84, 95, 97-105

scepticism 6, 51, 70-4, 79-81, 101
slippery slope 43-5, 75, 103-4,
   109-12
soul 3, 11, 13, 92
systemic death 4

transplantation 6, 21-2, 39, 45, 53,
   60-2, 65-6, 68, 71-2, 74-5, 89-90,
   95, 103-8

vegetative states 5-6, 8, 43-6, 84, 94,
   100, 107-8, 110-12
vitalism 80-1